W0043277

PRACTICAL PSYCHIATRY FOR THE HEALTH PROFESSIONAL

PRACTICAL PSYCHIATRY FOR THE HEALTH PROFESSIONAL

BY

CARLOS E. CLIMENT, M.D.
DEPARTMENT OF PSYCHIATRY
UNIVERSITY OF VALLE
CALI, COLUMBIA

AND

BARBARA J. BURNS, PH.D.
CHIEF, CLINICAL SERVICES RESEARCH BRANCH
DIVISION OF BIOMETRY AND EPIDEMIOLOGY
NATIONAL INSTITUTE OF MENTAL HEALTH
ROCKVILLE, MARYLAND

AND

DEPARTMENT OF PSYCHOLOGY
GRADUATE SCHOOL
HOOD COLLEGE
FREDERICK, MARYLAND

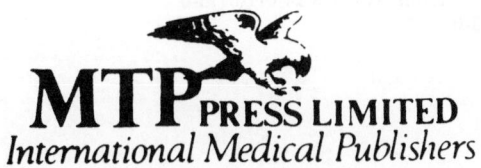

MTP PRESS LIMITED
International Medical Publishers

Published in the UK and Europe by
MTP Press Limited
Falcon House
Lancaster, England

Published in the US by
SPECTRUM PUBLICATIONS, INC.
175-20 Wexford Terrace
Jamaica, NY 11432

Copyright © 1984 by Spectrum Publications, Inc.
Softcover reprint of the hardcover 1st edition 1984
All rights reserved . No part of this book may be
reproduced in any form, by photostat, microfilm,
retrieval system, or any other means without prior
written permission of the copyright holder or his
licensee.

ISBN-13: 978-94-011-6715-4   e-ISBN-13: 978-94-011-6713-0
DOI: 10.1007/978-94-011-6713-0

DEDICATION

To Carlos Climent Caudet and to Robert Burns,
lives dedicated to effectively challenging established
systems.

Foreword

There is now widespread recognition that emotional problems, to say nothing of the interactions of emotions with other manifestations of illness and disease, constitute a substantial component of all human suffering. For too long the provision of medical care has been restricted to the physical aspects of that suffering while the psychological aspects have been shunned. Whether through ignorance about the nature of emotional illness and its clinical management, or through uncertainty about the legitimacy of their ministrations, physicians and many other health professionals have left the care of psychiatric problems to psychiatrists and other mental health professionals. For a variety of reasons this strategy is no longer feasible and substantial changes are required.

The extent of the needs, the nature of the presenting problems, the expectations of the patients, the prohibitive costs of alternative approaches, and the lack of trained mental health professionals make it imperative that general health workers learn to cope with the psychological and behavioral health problems of their patients. There are no other alternatives if the realities of comtemporary suffering, limited resources and psychobiological knowledge are accepted.

It is to the pragmatic knowledge base for this essential component of contemporary health care that this book makes a seminal contribution. Dr. Climent, from his experience both with educating young physicians and training support personnel to provide mental health services, and Dr. Burns, from her experience in providing and supervising those services bring a wealth of practical experience to bear on the preparation of this manual. They both have had extensive involvement with health professionals, patients and families at the level of primary health care where most mental health problems are seen initially and where they usually can be recognized and managed at the earliest and most tractable stages. In addition, the authors bring their experiences with both adults and children and, of course, families, to bear on their observations and recommendations.

The net result of their joint experiences is an eminently practical manual that can be readily understood by general health care professionals without specific psychiatric training. The authors skillfully relate the traditional "medical model" (which continues to shape most of the education of health professionals and most health services) to the realities of the behavioral and functional world that most people experience most of the time. The straightforward descriptions of presenting emotional states, the diagnostic algorithms and the practice strategies for clinical management provided by the authors should go a long way towards making most general medical professionals comfortable and competent in dealing with these problems.

Although textbooks of psychiatry for psychiatrists, and even textbooks of psychological medicine for general physicians, will continue to have a role in broadening our understanding of the complexities of mental illness, it is practical manuals such as this that make the amelioration of these problems an immediate, practical possibility. If all health professionals applied the knowledge and wisdom embodied in this volume, we would, indeed, approach the reality of making psychiatry practical for all those who can benefit from its insights and skills.

Kerr L. White, M.D.
The Rockefeller Foundation
New York, NY

Preface

Practical Psychiatry for the Health Professional provides the essentials for the diagnosis and clinical management of the most common psychiatric problems of adults and children seen by health professionals. Due to the realities of their work, health practitioners face the largest proportion of ambulatory psychiatric cases in any given community and thus constitute a most valuable, although largely underutilized, resource for the mentally ill. One of the reasons for this underutilization is the absence of appropriate guidelines for effective diagnosis, treatment and referral. Thus, clinicians avoid working in a field in which the diagnosis is perceived as ambiguous and the treatment process as unclear, complex and full of hypothetical alternatives. This manual attempts to tackle these issuses by presenting a training tool and a practical guide for daily work through simple but reliable mechanisms for diagnosis and a systematic approach to the management of the most common mental disorders seen in general medical practice.

Contents

SECTION 3—Clinical Problems in Children

Acknowledgments

We wish to thank: Maria Victoria de Arango, M.D., Universidad del Valle, Cali, Colombia, for her contribution of Chapters 1 and 3 and for her comments and suggestions throughout the entire manuscript; James W. Thompson, M.D., M.P.H., of the National Institute of Mental Health, U.S.A., for bringing his clinical, teaching, and research background to the writing of chapters 2 and 4 and for contributing a further psychiatric perspective through reviewing the remaining chapters; Cecilia Cordoba de Vargas, M.D., Child Psychiatrist at the El Paso Guidance Center in Texas, and Elizabeth Anne Gwaltney, M.A., of Frederick, Maryland, for reviewing and commenting on the child chapters; and Dorothea Bodison for her careful editing and patient revising and typing of many drafts of the manuscript.

PRACTICAL PSYCHIATRY FOR THE HEALTH PROFESSIONAL

Introduction

This manual is the product of the experience of a number of years of work in the primary care mental health field. It is a psychiatric manual for the diagnosis and treatment of the most common disorders in primary health care and is oriented toward the health professional. The model presented here views the general health professional as the front-line practitioner faced with the tasks of diagnosis and treatment of mental disorders, as well as the supervision of the technical support personnel (a complementary manual for the latter group was prepared by Carlos Climent and Maria Victoria de Arango and published by the Pan American Health Organization in 1983).

Traditional psychiatric textbooks for medical and nursing personnel tend to cover an exhaustive variety of mental disorders. The methods utilized for diagnosis often require considerable training and do not necessarily use objective methods for evaluation of different clinical syndromes. With regard to treatment, the guidelines offered are often excessive and vague, leaving the clinician with many unanswered decisions for which specialized training in clinical psychiatry also is required. Since, unfortunately, the latter situation seldom occurs, the consequence is that a significant group of health professionals prefer not to work with psychiatric patients.

The need for a practical manual for the diagnosis and treatment of the most common mental disorders by the general health professional provided the motivation for this text. We have attempted to design a manual in which sufficient and complete instructions for diagnosis are included without being unnecessarily complicated, with practical but not overly simplified guidelines covering important priorities in clinical practice. In addition, material is presented in a sequence that follows the thinking that the clinician would pursue when confronted with a person who suffers from a mental disorder. This should allow a diagnostic conclusion after excluding other important diagnostic con-

1

siderations, and should then be followed by a clear management plan. With straightforward guidelines for diagnosis and treatment, we hope that the resistance traditionally found in medicine toward psychiatry can be reduced. The principles guiding the development of these concepts are that psychiatric disorders can be diagnosed in objective, valid, and replicable ways, and that the therapeutic process can progress through a series of logical steps.

What is presented in this volume includes only selected psychiatric priorities for which a treatment program is possible at the primary health care level. The content of the chapters has been influenced by teaching clinical psychiatry to medical students at the Universidad del Valle, Cali, Colombia, and by the provision of mental health services in a neighborhood health center of the Massachusetts General Hospital in Boston as well as by research in this area conducted by both authors and others in the field.

The phenomenological emphasis in the diagnostic process is evident. For most disorders, the diagnostic criteria are to some extent based on the *Diagnostic and Statistical Manual of Mental Disorders*, Third Edition (DSM-III) of the American Psychiatric Association, published in 1980. The standard diagnostic questionnaires used in certain chapters have been adapted for clinical use from the Diagnostic Interview Schedule (DIS), a scale based on the DSM-III and designed by Lee N. Robins, Ph.D., and colleagues of Washington University in St. Louis, Missouri, under contract with the National Institute of Mental Health. One of the advantages offered by the questionnaires is the possibility of making a diagnosis on the basis of a simple, standardized approach. Even though the DIS was designed to produce diagnoses in epidemiological studies, the modifications suggested in this volume constitute an attempt to use it as a clinical instrument.

Other diagnostic questionnaires, as well as the flow charts, had been designed as a supplement to training programs for physicians and nurses offered since 1976 by the Department of Psychiatry, Universidad del Valle, Cali, Colombia. In their preliminary versions, certain diagnostic flow charts were used in the World Health Organization Collaborative Study on Strategies to Extend Mental Health Services. The management flow charts constitute a summary of clinical judgments. The clinical approach presented, which utilizes questionnaires and diagnostic and management flow charts, also provides the potential for close and efficient supervision at each step in the clinical process.

The orientation regarding treatment is eclectic with an emphasis on supportive therapies and psychopharmacological knowledge. Many nosological entities are excluded due to their low frequency or because their complex management procedures are unlikely to occur within the daily activities of a busy general medical clinician. In other instances, we decided to exclude certain disorders because of the lack of a known effective treatment for these conditions at the present time.

The reader will observe differences in the coverage of the different syndromes. For example, the phenomenological aspects of psychosis are treated extensively, whereas other syndromes are covered only briefly. This decision was based on previous teaching experiences. Also, some chapters cover problems such as agitation, which are not considered diagnostic categories but are problems which require clinical knowledge on the part of the general practitioner. Other differences in the diagnostic and management flowcharts or in the presence of additional tables for the differential diagnosis are due to the specific requirements of knowledge or skills for each condition.

We recognize the difficulties facing the innovative nature of this manual and are prepared to measure its usefulness through its ability to generate new ideas and to assess its flexibility to adapt to different clinical settings.

1.
Approaches to Interviewing and Evaluation

CHAPTER 1

Principles of Interviewing

MARIA VICTORIA DE ARANGO, M.D.

The purpose of the medical/psychiatric interview is to gain knowledge about the patient and to make a diagnosis that will determine a treatment process. What type of information do we want to obtain from our patients? We will certainly want to obtain data about the patient's illness, but it is also necessary to acquire information about the patient's perception of his surroundings, his attitudes towards life, his expectations, values, fears, strengths, interests, and also his own understanding of what is happening to him. All of this is absolutely necessary in order to treat the patient as an individual, not an illness, and as a whole human being.

It has been emphasized when teaching students in the health field, and more so in the past decade, that the interview is fundamental to the diagnostic process. Early in their training, medical students are told that 90% of the diagnosis is obtained through the clinical history which is the result of an effective and reliable interview.

Parallel to these teachings, the student has been gaining knowledge about data obtained through the physical examination and laboratory tests, and frequently begins to rely more heavily on this quantitative information, as opposed to the verbal account obtained from the patient through the interview. Frequently, the trainee begins to feel that the patient's account of his symptoms is inadequate and unreliable and that the only "good and trustworthy" information comes from the physician's direct physical examination and from "hard" data obtained through laboratory tests. Consequently, the ability to use these "hard" data is seen as the most valued skill to be learned, and more time is spent by students practicing to identify physical signs of illness, than to obtain a patient's history or to observe and identify the data reported and emotions expressed by their patients.

Furthermore, the student is placed in a setting where the reliance on "hard" data is reinforced. His observation of the practices of staff physicians and his teachers, who often devote more time and concern to the physical and laboratory examinations and their results than to verbal exchange and human interaction with their patients, serves to convince the student that history taking is merely a task to be completed as quickly as possible.

It is the purpose of this chapter to present some of the theory behind this often-neglected area of the interview. The purpose of the interview is the same for all clinical areas, be it surgery, internal medicine or psychiatry, and in recent years more attention has been placed on the principles and techniques with regard to the medical/psychiatric interview as it relates to the interviewing process in the entire health field. Bearing this in mind, it is important to review some salient aspects of the medical/psychiatric interview that are relevant to all physicians and therapists of the health field.

FACTORS THAT AFFECT THE PHYSICIAN-PATIENT RELATIONSHIP

A good relationship is essential to the practice of medicine. Patients believe that physicians, especially psychiatrists, are capable of handling even the most difficult life situations and can be trusted with all kinds of information. But even with this positive start, patients need to be treated as individuals and will respond with more in-depth and reliable information when there is a trusting relationship with the physician. One basic element in the development of a good relationship is the establishment of rapport, defined as a conscious, genuine responsiveness between physician and patient. In addition to good rapport, another basic element in the interview situation is that of transference. Transference is the emotional response of the patient toward the health professional, and is based on the patient's needs, fears, and earlier experiences or conflicts. A psychiatrist may use transference as a therapeutic tool in the performance of psychotherapy. The primary care provider usually does not, but needs to be aware of this phenomenon and use it to positive advantage in relating to the patient.

The health professional will also have feelings about the patient, called "countertransference." Here the psychotherapist and primary health care provider have the same responsibility, that is, to recognize these "counter feelings," and to avoid allowing them to interfere with the patient's care. For instance, the provider may find himself or herself very angry at a patient, even though the patient has done little to elicit such anger. On reflection, the provider may be able to identify a previous experience, reminiscent of the present situation, during which he or she became angry. It would, then, be inappropriate to express anger in the present situation. The major thing that can alert the provider to "counter feelings" is the presence of a strong emotion that is out of proportion to the stimulus from the patient.

THE PHYSICIAN'S ROLE

There are no strict guidelines for the behavior of a physician in regard to his patients. The specific style of interaction that the physician adopts is something that evolves individually through direct verbal communication with patients and to some extent depends on his own personality patterns. Important in the development of his own personal style is reading about and studying interviewing techniques, and observing videotapes and live interviews. The young physician can then continue to develop his own style through interviews with patients. This is the most difficult task undertaken by the trainee and no other activity can be substituted for it. The medical/psychiatric interview often poses the greatest difficulty for medical students and young physicians, due to the massive expression of emotions and unexpected or strange attitudes that may be expressed by their patients. Handling these situations can be a trying experience if students are not given an opportunity to explore their own emotions, fears and shortcomings in regard to the contact with patients and in regard to their own, sometimes idealized, version of what constitutes a successful physician.

Some concerns expressed by advanced medical students after several interviews with mentally ill patients are the following:

I was so worried about asking the right questions that I didn't even listen to what the patient was trying to tell me.

I felt a complete failure when the patient started asking me personal questions. I felt I was no longer in control and couldn't decide whether to ignore or answer the questions.

I expected hostile or aggressive behavior at any moment and couldn't concentrate on what the patient was saying.

When I asked questions about delusions and hallucinations, I felt it was not relevant to the patient and felt embarrassed.

I suddenly ran out of prepared questions and the patient and I were silent for a long time. I couldn't think of anything else to say, it was very uncomfortable.

The learning process must deal with many concerns such as these so that the student interviewer can develop the most beneficial and therapeutic relationship with his patients. If the physician is aware of and comfortable with his own abilities, concerns, fears, and shortcomings, he will be confident and spontaneous with his patients. Such an attitude will then lead to a more successful therapeutic relationship.

The physician's interest in his patient is not necessarily shown exclusively through verbal expression but also through attitudes communicated. The physician's interest is evidenced in the attention given to what the patient is saying, by exploring the meaning of what the patient has expressed, and by answering the patient's most urgent questions to the best of his ability.

Acceptance of patients is an important, although not necessarily easy achievement. Some patients may be irritating or unattractive to the physician, hold conflicting beliefs or views about important issues, or disclose shocking situations. If the physician does not take advantage of his position as an expert in order to try to change behaviors that are not relevant to the patient's health, his ability to communicate with many difficult patients may improve. He should not feel that irritating or aggressive comments from his patients are directed at him personally, but rather that they may constitute a revival of previous experiences. Therefore, aggression should not be responded to with aggression, but rather by trying to allay the fears and mistrust in the patient, which are frequently the cause for such behaviors. Moral judgments, either through verbal expressions or gestures, are also contraindicated as a response to confidential information provided by the patient.

PATIENT ATTITUDES

The patient's attitudes towards the physician will be determined in part by relationships with earlier authoritative figures, these attitudes may include emotional responses, preconceived ideas, expectations, fears, and, in the best of cases, calm and trust.

Undesirable, however, is the idealized image of the omnipotent physician who will resolve all of the patient's troubles without any effort on the patient's part. To deal with this idealized image, the physician can, for example, avoid the temptation to calm a patient with regard to the severity or implications of the illness before he has gained an adequate knowledge of the patient's illness, even though the patient may appear to be very vulnerable. A more realistic relationship and more beneficial results will be gained by assuring the patient of the physician's interest in learning in depth about the illness and giving adequate treatment to the best of his ability.

COMMUNICATION

Even though the physician and patient may speak the same language, misunderstandings can result from the assumption that words have definite and rigid meanings for all. The inexperienced interviewer may lack the skills and initiative to explore the patient's comments, and this will impede a thorough exploration and adequate insight into the patient's problems. If the physician seems not to hear what the patient is saying, the patient may resent the physician's apparent incapacity to understand what he is trying to express and may feel that he cannot be helped.

In addition to exploring the patient's comments, the patient's cultural context, education, and beliefs should be known in order to gain accurate information that will help establish a diagnosis and help in the patient's treatment. Such an understanding will also enable the physician to express himself in such a way that the patient understands at all times what he needs to know about his illness, allowing him to follow the physician's precise recommendations.

THE INITIAL INTERVIEW

Most patients are anxious when they consult a physician and have difficulty expressing their complaints. The physician's provision of a private and quiet atmosphere lessens the initial anxiety of the patient and fosters his confidence. The physician's attitude should be respectful but not distant or hurried; the patient should know that even though the physician's time is limited, during the interview he will have his undivided attention.

The traditional, and probably best way to initiate an interview is for the physician to introduce himself and then ask the patient about the reason for his visit, allowing the patient to express his complaint freely; in other words, the patient is encouraged to "tell his own story." Pertinent exploratory questions should be asked by the physician, trying to use the patient's own words when describing his problems. This makes the questions far more relevant to the patient. When the patient realizes that the physician will not pass judgment or ridicule him, this will act to motivate the patient to express his problems more fully. This is especially true when giving accounts of sexual or aggressive behaviors.

The physician should be flexible and allow for a natural rhythm within the interview, whether the topic is serious or trivial. For example, without abandoning his professional and respectful attitude, he can permit himself to enjoy a humorous situation along with his patient. Again, interest, flexibility, and comprehension are determinants of a successful intervention.

Formulating and Organizing Questions

Once the emotional climate of the interview has been achieved and the initial complaints have been expressed by the patient, the physician should be vigilant to make appropriate interventions. He can use the patient's own words to expand concepts. While inviting the patient to freely present his own concerns, the health professional should by no means adopt a passive role and can guide the spontaneous flow of the interview towards areas that need further exploration.

While short silent periods are acceptable and can be used by the physician and also by the patient to revise and organize the materials, long silences that tend to make the patient uncomfortable should be avoided. Open-ended questions are preferable in order to avoid yes-no answers. The avoidance of technical language facilitates the comprehension by and the response of the patient.

Another way in which the physician can stimulate new thoughts in the patient, or help the patient to understand his own emotional responses, is to make an "interpretation." This consists of condensing and organizing several of the patient's comments and/or emotional reactions, and reflecting his formulation to the patient. Although this kind of interpretation is not at the same depth at which a psychiatrist may work, nevertheless it can help the patient discover new possibilities in regard to his illness. Even if no new insights are reached by the patient, such an intervention shows the patient that the health professional is genuinely interested, and fosters further sharing of information.

Terminating the Interview

Although most primary care interviews will be shorter, an interview should not exceed an hour or ninety minutes at the most. Fatigue or excessive strain in the patient are indications of the need to end the interview. Informing the patient of the approaching end of the interview a few minutes before allows him to finish his comments and to introduce any additional information. A preliminary evaluation by the physician of what has been said facilitates the development of plans for future interviews.

REFERENCES

Bird B. *Talking with Patients*, 2nd Ed. Philadelphia: Lippincott, 1973.
Enelow AJ, Swisher SN. *Interviewing and Patient Care*, 2nd Ed. New York: Oxford University Press, 1979.

CHAPTER 2

Therapeutic Communication

JAMES W. THOMPSON, M.D., M.P.H.

This chapter deals with practical approaches to problems in communication, and makes the basic point that an HP who does not take into account the psychosocial aspects of the patient's illness places himself or herself in a technician's role. Since psychological, social, cultural, familial, economic and spiritual needs of patients interact with biological ones, it is essential to develop relationships with patients which facilitate the communication of the preceding kinds of concerns. It is illustrated that in any contact with a patient there is a potential relationship, which can be used positively or negatively.

POTENTIAL RELATIONSHIPS

The existence of a relationship between the patient and yourself is one which at first may seem to exist a priori. The roles of "doctor" and "patient" have meanings in any society that call forth the image of a particular kind of relationship, and the same is true of any member of the health care team. Closer examination of this "relationship" often reveals that, although interactions occur between two persons, still only a *potential* relationship exists. Even when a relationship does exist, it may be ineffective or dysfunctional. Several guiding principles to make a potential relationship into a therapeutic tool follow.

Engage the Patient as a Person.

You may well do this already. But even the most empathetic and humanistic HP must constantly be on guard that the patient isn't seen merely as a vector for his or her pathogen. Even our terminology points this out, as we (for example) may refer to a patient named Ms. Jones as "a diabetic," as though this explains everything important there is to know about Ms. Jones (and all the Ms. Joneses who "are diabetics"). There are some obvious ways to engage a patient, such as calling the patient by name, making eye contact with the patient, and allowing the patient to exercise appropriate modesty during examinations. Another way to engage the patient is to avoid talking about the patient as though he or she were not there. A consultation by the bedside, with the patient present, is inappropriate *unless* the patient is a part of the discussion.

Use nontechnical language. Most patients want to understand what you are saying, and when spoken to in their native language will understand much more than most HPs give them credit for. Saying "you wouldn't understand" is a good way to insure noncompliance.

Use examples to let patients know what is happening to them. Be "folksy" if you do this well, but don't "talk down" to a patient. Your style will vary from patient to patient, of course. Do not gear your explanations to a patient's socioeconomic or sociocultural group alone, but rather to his or her individual level of sophistication. Also, to ensure that the patient understands your explanation, double-check, taking responsibility for your explanation. ("Am I being clear about this?" is *much* better than "Are you able to understand this?").

Give the Patient Space.

One way to block a relationship with a patient is by "crowding" the patient. This may be done by rushing the patient or by filling every silent period with questions or chatter. Give the patient "space" to talk to you. If the patient seems to be waiting for a "cue" from you, let him/her know that he or she has your attention by saying, "Has anything been going on that we need to talk about?"

Another way to crowd patients is to give them only hurried time. Some HPs can spend half an hour with a patient and seem rushed the entire time. Others can spend ten minutes and give the impression of not being hurried at all. Patients of the first HP will feel rushed in half an hour, while patients of the second may feel quite satisfied that they were listened to. The key is to provide "good" time—unhurried, empathetic, and productive time—rather than necessarily providing a *lot* of time. "Good" time can also be efficient. A patient might go through three visits with a "crowding" physician or nurse practitioner before the real problem emerges, while one visit would be enough with "good" time.

Avoid Pressure In Gathering Data.

In the training of health care professionals there is enormous emphasis placed on gathering clinical data as quickly as possible. Unfortunately this tends to focus the interaction on "what the doctor or nurse wants to know," rather than on "what the patient wants to convey." Patients, if given a chance, will often give information and convey concerns directly. They may, however, use the following clues, which must be listened for carefully:

- spoken clues (e.g., "I feel *pretty* good today")
- unspoken clues (e.g., what is pointedly left out)
- anxiety, sadness, anger, and other emotional reactions
- periods of silence
- eye contact ("meaningful looks," or lack of eye contact)
- body language (e.g., shifting about, gripping the arm of the chair, "curled up" body posture).

EXAMPLE: Consider the case of a 13-year-old girl named Joyce:

Doctor: "Hello Joyce, what seems to be the trouble today?"
Patient: "I have a sore throat."
Doctor: "How long has it been sore?"
Patient: "About a week."
Doctor: "Any other symptoms? Fever, chills, and the like?"
Patient: "No, not exactly." [the clue]
Doctor: "Not exactly?" [here the physician gives a clear message to the patient to go on and say what is on her mind]

Watch for the "Ticket of Admission."

Patients frequently have several reasons for coming to see the HP. The "presenting complaint" may be real enough, but this also may serve as a "ticket" to see you for another reason. If the patient finds you to be interested, empathetic, and someone to be trusted, and if you watch and respond to the "clues" described above, a second and more important (at least to the patient) issue may emerge. The "sore throat" in the example above could be considered a "ticket of admission."

Hold Self-Disclosure In Respect and Confidence.

Once patients disclose something about themselves that is important to them, it is necessary for the HP to adopt a respectful posture towards this self-disclosure. The patient usually fears that you:

- will laugh at him (or her)
- will think he's bad

- will think he's crazy
- will tell his wife (husband, mother, father, or other significant person)

It is important to avoid doing the above and to provide reassurance concerning these fears. If the patient openly asks whether you think he is bad, crazy, or whether you will tell his secret to a significant person, the course of action is clear. You simply provide the reassurance. A reluctant patient, however, will have to be encouraged.

EXAMPLE: Ms. Smith, a 45-year-old white woman, has told the physician's assistant (P.A.) that she wants to reveal something, then lapses into silence.

    P.A.: "You said you wanted to tell me something."
    Patient: "Yes, well . . . I don't know, really."
    P.A.: "Is something stopping you?"
    Patient: [nods affirmatively]
    P.A.: "Maybe you're afraid I will think badly of you."
    Patient: "Well, no, you've been very kind."
    P.A.: "So this is a secret, perhaps?"
    Patient: "Yes."
    P.A.: "And you wouldn't want your family members to know?"
    Pateint: "Especially my daughter."
    P.A.: "Don't let that worry you. I won't divulge your secret to your daughter unless you tell me I can."
    Patient: [Goes on to tell her secret].

One thing that will become apparent is that the secrets of most patients are not as terrible as the patients think they are. You may, however, learn things that you feel you need to share with a colleague. This is why the P.A. above kept his promise to a specific person, avoiding a promise not to tell anyone at all about Ms. Smith's secret. If he had been pressed for a total promise of confidentiality (which rarely happens), he could say, "If someone's secret has legal implications, I occasionally have to tell someone. Otherwise, I will not reveal your secret unless you tell me I can."

Deal with Feelings.

It is not enough to deal with "the problem" intellectually. Patients have feelings about their illnesses and other difficulties. That you will allow them to cry or to show anger may be quite important to their willingness to let you be of help to them.

Send the Patient Home with Something.

Properly or improperly, patients often want to leave the doctor's office "with something." Untold gallons of penicillin have been given inappropriately because of this phenomenon. Part of the answer to this dilemma is to have all patients leave with one or more of the following:

- a careful evaluation of both their presenting complaint *and* other significant problems
- a feeling of having been listened to as a person and having been treated with respect
- a feeling of having gotten "it" off their chest
- even if no solution is forthcoming, at least a promise from you to work with them towards a solution or an appropriate referral to a source of help.

One thing that is tempting to give the patient is advice about personal problems. This is not wise, however. If you give advice that works, the patient may see this as something *you* did, rather than something he or she did him/herself. If your advice doesn't work, your credibility with the patient may suffer. Rather, define your role as someone who will listen, suggest alternatives, and assist the patient in reaching his/her own solutions to a given problem.

SPECIAL PROBLEMATIC PATIENTS

In dealing with patients, there are many special situations that can be helped or hindered by the quality of the therapeutic relationship. Several will be discussed here: the angry patient; the seductive patient; the demanding patient; the inquisitive patient; and the silent patient.

The Angry Patient

Anger is difficult to deal with, especially when it is directed at you. There are some ways to have anger work for the best interests of the therapeutic process, however.

- Don't take it personally. Even if you're a source of the anger in a very real way, chances are that there are multiple determinants, many of which have nothing to do with you personally. (See "transference" in Chapter 1, "Principles of Interviewing," pp. 7-12). Adopt the stance that you're glad the patient trusts you enough to share the anger with you.
- Recognize the anger. Saying "I understand that you're really angry" immediately puts you into alliance with the patient. Then saying, "I'd like to

understand more about why you're angry" is a fine second step.

- If you can help, do so. If you can't help, explain why.
- You can accept the reason for the anger, even if you don't agree. Saying "I can understand why you're angry" doesn't commit you to the patient's position. You can even make this more overt by saying, "I can't say that I completely agree, but I can understand why you might be angry about that."
- If you feel that you're about to lose your temper, say "I don't think we're getting anywhere right now. I'm going to leave for a few minutes, then I'll be back and we can continue our discussion." Or, "This is a very important issue. Let's set aside some time later in the week to discuss it further."

These techniques may not work if the patient is suffering from certain mental disorders. Among these are mania, some organic brain syndromes, and paranoid psychosis. If the anger seems not to respond to such interventions as illustrated, consult Chapter 11, "Psychosis" and Chapter 7, "Organic Brain Syndromes." If the patient seems acutely out of control, do not argue with him or her and do obtain psychiatric help.

The Seductive Patient

The relationship between you and the patient is a close one. That is, you are working on something very important together—the patient's health. At times a patient may wish this relationship to be an intimate one. This may be stated as "being friends" with no sexual connotation, or may be overtly sexual. Intimacy is, of course, never appropriate, unless the professional-patient relationship has been terminated. To handle such a situation without rejecting the patient as a person, try the following:

- Don't be seductive yourself, even jokingly. Watch the thin line between friendliness and flirtation.
- Have a chaperone with you in potentially "loaded" situations, or leave the door to the office open.
- If the seductive behavior has never occurred before, and it isn't too overt, you might simply ignore it. Most patients take the hint.
- If the patient persists or is very overt, don't be angry or rejecting, but recognize the situation in a matter-of-fact way. ("I somehow get the idea that you are expecting more of our relationship than one between doctor or nurse and a patient.")
- Clarify things, even if the patient denies his or her seductiveness. "I need you to know that I'm glad to be your doctor or nurse, but I do not mix private and professional relationships." This can be said in a matter-of-fact voice, not in a rejecting or hostile way.

●Don't give the patient a lecture. Let him or her save face. (Besides, he or she may not have been aware of seductive behavior.)

The Demanding Patient

Some patients demand a lot, sometimes appropriately. Some, however, demand too much, too often. When they do, try these suggestions:

●Be clear in your own mind about how far you will go. (For example, you may be willing to write a note to the patient's boss, but not to call the boss.)
●Communicate clearly to the patient what you will and will not do (again, matter-of-factly, not in a hostile way).
●Explain the reason for your position if you wish, but don't feel that you *have* to explain, e.g., "I'm aware that you don't understand completely why I won't do that, but that is a position I feel I must maintain.
●Beware of becoming "the bad guy." Assertions such as "you don't care" should be met with calm denial and restatement of your limits. Your own anger and defensiveness may tend to place you into a "bad-guy" role. Simply refuse to play this role by not becoming angry or defensive.
●Accept the patient's anger and disappointment if these emotions are expressed. You can always choose to understand empathetically.
●Give the demanding patient alternatives to choose from (all of which you are willing to do). This lets the patient have some control over what happens, but still maintains your boundaries. ("What I would be willing to do is write your boss a note, have him call me with you present in his office, or send him a report of my examination. Tell me which you would prefer.")

The Inquisitive Patient

Patients will frequently want to know personal things about you. You do not have an obligation to answer questions you do not feel comfortable with, however. For instance, you may be willing to say that you are married, but may not want to discuss your spouse. There are several ways to deal with a patient who wants personal data from you.

●One way is to say, "I realize that you are interested in knowing about me, but we have only a very short time to deal with your problem and we need to spend our time doing that."
●Another way is to turn the question back to the patient.

EXAMPLE: Dr. Vasquez is interviewing Mr. Brown.

Patient: "How is your wife, doctor?"
Doctor: "Fine, and how is your family?"

Patient: "Okay . . . Do you have children, doctor?"
Doctor: "Yes . . . You have a 5-year-old that was in last week. How is she?"
Patient: "Well, doctor, she's still pretty sick." [etc.]

●If the patient is very insistent and you are uncomfortable giving out the requested information, it is perfectly appropriate to say, "I'm really not willing to discuss that." (This is not said in an angry way, but rather in an "informational" manner.)

Always bear in mind, however, that such questions frequently do not really have to do with you. Rather, as in the example, they may be the patient's way of bringing up an issue of importance.

The Silent Patient

Perhaps one of the most frustrating experiences in medical/psychiatric interviewing is the patient who will not talk to you. If this occurs, consider the following:

●Is this a "clue," such as is described above?
●Is the patient in a new environment, which he/she finds intimidating?
●Does the patient not speak your language?
●Is the patient profoundly depressed?
●Is the patient aphasic?
●Is the patient a child or teenager who is scared or angry about being where he or she is?
●Is the patient mute because of a psychosis? [unusual]

If depression or psychosis is suspected, refer to the appropriate chapter in this book (Chapter 5, "The Syndrome of Depression," or Chapter 11, "Psychosis"). If the patient is scared, intimidated, or angry, understanding and reassurance are indicated. If language is the problem, a translator can be obtained. If the origin of the patient's silence remains unclear and you do not have time to spend trying to solve the riddle, a psychiatric referral may be helpful.

There is one time when silence can be "golden." This is when you are counseling a patient on a personal problem. A measured amount of silence can convey the message, "I am interested in what you have to say and am willing to give you enough time to think about what you want to say, and to feel the things you need to feel." This is not to say that you should be a "blank screen." Signs that you are listening to the patient, whether this is a nod of the head, an "uh-huh," or other facilitating comments, are quite appropriate.

CONCLUSION

The point of this chapter is not to teach the HP to be a psychotherapist, or even a counselor. Such training is long and involved and is beyond the scope of this book. Rather, the intent is to help the HP improve his or her communication techniques with each patient he or she sees. Such techniques are useful with any patient, whether the problem is an upper respiratory infection, congestive heart failure, or a depressive disorder. Each patient encounter will be greatly strengthened when such therapeutic communication has taken place.

REFERENCES

Hall RCW (Ed.). *Psychiatric Presentations of Medical Illness: Somatopsychic Disorders.* New York: Spectrum, 1980.

Kimsey, LR, Roberts JL. *Referring the Psychiatric Patient: A Guide for the Physician.* Springfield, Ill.: Charles C. Thomas, 1973.

Walker S III. *Psychiatric Signs and Symptoms Due to Medical Problems.* Springfield, Ill.: Charles C. Thomas, 1967.

Wittkower ED, Warnes H. *Psychosomatic Medicine: Its Clinical Applications.* Hagerstown, Md.: Harper and Row, 1977.

CHAPTER 3

The History

MARIA VICTORIA DE ARANGO, M.D.

In the traditional medical model, the information obtained in the medical/
psychiatric interview is divided into two sections: the patient's history and
the mental status.* This chapter discusses the former. The psychiatric portion of the history explores characteristics that are of a more subjective nature
and therefore far more difficult to explore than the portion of the medical
history that details somatic complaints. Consequently, it is essential to master
a partially nondirective technique, which will permit the patient to "tell his
own story" while still allowing for the specific exploration of areas regarded
as important by the clinician.

The purpose of obtaining the clinical history is to give the health professional (HP) the information that will help him understand his patient. This
information will deal with the patient's development, environment, and adap-
tive mechanisms. It will also include data about the patient's home and relatives, his occupation and education. This information should provide a clear
indication of the patient's functioning before the illness.

If allowed to do so, the patient will present his most urgent concerns to
the HP. These may not, however, be the first concerns presented. It is the HP's
responsibility to receive, organize, and expand this material in order to obtain
a clear description of the chief complaint and present illness. The importance
of an accurate, well-recorded clinical history can never be emphasized enough.
This constitutes an invaluable source of information to increase the HP's understanding of the patient's problems.

_____

*Because this book may be used by some early in their training, the basics of a
clinical history are included here. The practicing clinician may find it useful as
a review.

The psychiatric clinical history has been divided into the following sections: identification data; chief complaint; present illness; personal history; family history; and personality.

Identification of the Patient

This includes the patient's name, age, sex, marital status, education, occupation, and present address. This information is crucial for follow-up, statistics, and scientific studies. Some clinical uses of such information are to give an indication of possible support from the family; to point to specific syndromes (e.g., those that are age-related); or to indicate inadequate physical or mental development.

Chief Complaint

It is important to state the complaint in the patient's own words. Frequently, more technical information may seem more important from the psychiatric/ medical viewpoint. Nevertheless, the patient's chief concern should not be taken lightly and should be explored. To do so will strengthen the patient's trust in the clinician. The patient's initial comments constitute his perception of the problem to be discussed and can be used as a baseline from which to evaluate changes at later stages of treatment.

Present Illness

This is in essence the patient's story. At this stage, the HP's patience and interest often will be put to the test, as she/he frequently will have expectations of what the patient should say and in what order. However, the patient has "lived" the illness, not studied it, and consequently, the account often is not a coherent, organized, chronological statement, complete with precipitating factors. Although the patient expresses himself adequately in regard to those symptoms or situations that trouble him the most, he may minimize or plainly ignore other symptoms, emotions, or situations that have coexisted and that are crucial.

It is, of course, up to the clinician to listen to and understand the patient's complaint and to expand this information through probing questions, formulating the patient's report into chronological order. Not only should the events be explored, but also the motivations and emotions related to them. Such factors are frequently ignored by relatives or informants. It is important to determine if this is the first such episode presented by the patient; if there have been previous episodes, it is necessary to explore the characteristics of each of them, the treatment of each of them, the treatment given, and the outcome. Precipitating family, personal, and environmental factors should be explored. The patient should be asked how he became ill and what it has meant to him and his family. Treatments for previous episodes may be explored in consultation with other clinicians, should they be available.

A practical question, which could help determine the onset of the patient's illness could be: "When was the last time you felt completely well?"

In the case of a patient who denies his problems completely or has great difficulty reporting them, a trustworthy informant, clearly identified with respect to his relationship to the patient over a certain period of time, should be interviewed to obtain the patient's clinical history.

Personal History

The patient's personal history refers to the stages of his development, the sociocultural context, the description of significant others and/or authority figures, and events related to these periods: infancy, childhood, adolescence and adulthood. Specific areas for exploration are outlined below.

Infancy

This period should be explored directly with the parents, if the patient is a child. Information regarding whether the pregnancy was planned, the presence of illness or drug treatments during pregnancy, and factors concerning labor and the neonatal period are all important. The first year of life should be investigated with regard to psychomotor development, nourishment, specific illnesses, excessive activity, the child's display of emotions, the relationship with parents and family, and the parents' satisfaction or dissatisfaction with the infant's specific behavior and development.

Childhood

The child's behavior and development from age one until adolescence should be explored, specifically with regard to illness and how it affected the patient and the family, psychomotor development (walking, toilet training, language development), as well as sleeping patterns (e.g., nightmares and fear of darkness).

Additional topics to explore are games the patient plays or played, his reaction to peers, and his interaction in groups. If there were significant changes in the environment or early loss of close family members, the child's reaction should be described.

Any behavior changes at entry into school should be described and, in addition, the patient's academic and social progress, along with hobbies and special interests should be explored. Display of emotions and affection in the family unit should be discussed. Reactions by the parents to sexual curiosity or sexual behaviors in the child should be explored, as well as their reaction to aggressive behaviors.

Adolescence

In this developmental period, certain areas of the patient's functioning deserve exploration in depth. During this period, many biological changes and social demands connected with puberty must be met. Closely associated with adolescence are behaviors that deal with self-assertion, choosing of goals, relating to the opposite sex, belonging to a group, handling external and internal feelings of aggression, and relating to adults. The health professional needs to be able to explore in an open and nonjudgmental manner such matters as the patient's reactions to biological and social changes such as the emergence of sexual impulses, body changes, fantasies, relationships with the opposite sex, and homosexual fantasies or behaviors. The adolescent's academic development, his relationship with peers, with teachers and with adults in general should also be explored, in addition to his parents' attitudes and reactions to these behaviors.

Adulthood

Although it is difficult to determine the exact onset of this period, we can consider as an appropriate definition the time when the individual is self-supporting, even though he may continue to live with parents or relatives. This exploration should deal with the individual's life goals, self-fulfillment, and whether his present occupation is satisfactory. The stability of the patient should be assessed in regard to work and adult relationships. If the patient is married, the reasons for his choice can be reviewed, together with the actual functioning of the marriage, children, and relationships with in-laws. Sexual relationships should be explored in depth in regard to satisfaction for both partners, whether they are orgasmic, and whether both are satisfied with the frequency and characteristics of intercourse.

Family History

The patient's parents and siblings should be described with regard to age, sex, occupation, and their relationship with the patient. It is important to determine whether the patient has idealized or realistic images of his family members. Illnesses in family members should be explored, in particular those dealing with mental disturbances, extreme aggressive behavior, alcoholism, and convulsive disorders.

Personality

The description of the personal history should have shed light on the patient's personality traits. Nevertheless, it is important to sum up certain salient characteristics that have been identified in the patient. These can also be clarified by asking further questions of the patient and of the relative and informants. One way to investigate this area would be for the patient to describe himself using single adjectives (such as "kind", "impatient," or "forceful"). Relatives and informants could be asked to do the same. This is a useful exercise that will help the physician to establish realistic goals in the treatment of this particular individual, and can also help the patient and relatives accept the limitations of this treatment.

Although assessing the patient's personality characteristics is an important part of the history, even the most successful therapeutic intervention seldom modify basic personality traits. Understanding something about these traits can, however, help the health professional be more effective in correcting maladaptive behavior patterns associated with nonpsychiatric organic illness and/or with mental disorder.

CHAPTER 4

The Mental Status Examination

JAMES W. THOMPSON, M.D., M.P.H.

Every patient should receive a short mental status exam, regardless of the presenting complaint. Other patients will need a longer exam. The organization of this chapter is intended to serve both purposes. A "complete" mental status exam is found on the left side of each page, while a summary is found on the right. Items on the right that are felt by the authors to be basic to any medical examination are marked with a crosshatch (#). Note that some items are observations by the clinician, while others require questioning the patient.

1. General Appearance and Relationship to the HP

Be alert to the patient's race and religion. Those could shed light on beliefs that should be considered when evaluating the patient.

What is patient's race?
What is his/her religion?   #

It should be stated whether the patient is clean and appropriately dressed or in disarray and conspicuous. The relationship to the HP may be described as collaborative, guarded, isolated, etc. Was the patient friendly or openly hostile? Was the patient alert and did he accept the interview situation?

Is the patient's dress appropriate?   #

Is the patient friendly, hostile, isolated, distant?   #

29

2. Motor Behavior

The clinician should describe the patient's motor behaviors during the interview and the appropriateness of them. Hyperactivity and slowness in movements should be noted. Extremely slow movements could be described as being in "slow motion." Qualitatively, the following are some of the more extreme motor behaviors displayed by patients:

Does the patient exhibit unusual movements?   #

a. repetitive involuntary motor behavior, characterized by purposeless movements, or actions performed in a repetitive manner that are significant only to the patient;

Repetitive movements?

b. fixed posture, where the patient adopts a certain position and does not move for long periods;

Fixed position?

c. bizarre behavior, which may include any manner that appears "crazy" or strange.

Bizarre behavior?

3. Emotional Reaction

Here the clinician should note the emotional reactions of the patient. They should be described as appropriate or inappropriate to the specific thought content being expressed. The patient's face and attitude can also be observed in order to ascertain that the emotions displayed are consistent with what is being verbally expressed.

Note the patient's emotional reactions.   #

Are emotions appropriate to the topic?   #

Some possible emotional reactions are sadness, euphoria, aggressiveness, hostility, silliness, childishness, bluntness, etc.

What emotion is being   #
expressed?

4. Thought Process

Evaluate changes in thought process or in the flow of thought. Disorders of the flow of thought have to do with faulty associa-

Is there a disorder of   #
thought?

tional structure and may be evidenced in how the patient expresses himself. These disorders may also be reflected by an abnormal thinking rate (i.e., excessively fast or slow). The goal-orientation of the thinking process may be lost, represented by flight of ideas, tangentiality, and clang associations. Some other frequent findings are neologisms, incoherence, and irrelevance.

"Loose associations"?

Rapid or slow speech?

(1) *Incoherence.* Verbal expressions are empty or obscure; the main idea cannot be determined, and no conclusions may be reached (e.g., "the value of such is much, not mush or lush").

Is there incoherence?

(2) *Neologisms.* The patient creates a completely new word or expression. (Neologisms frequently sound similar to the real words, but in fact they have meaning only to the patient, e.g., "Doctor, I have an *extrapropensiary* ability to the feeling of pain in my stomach.")

Are there new words (neologisms)?

(3) *"Flight of ideas"* is a rapid thinking rate wherein the patient cannot express verbally the ideas that come to his mind quickly enough, and therefore skips some ideas, loosening the associational bonds. Rapid speech will be noted.

Is "flight of ideas" present?

(4) *Tangentiality.* The patient answers the question by referring to the idea but not completely answering it. Frequently, the same question must be repeated in order to understand the answer. (For example, when the patient is asked for how long he/she has had a certain symptom, he/she may answer: "Well, I have been bothered by it and some other circumstances may have affected me.")

Does the patient give tangential answers?

(5) *Clang associations* occur when the associational bonds are determined by the *sound* of the words and are not goal-oriented (e.g., "He must think I was late, hate, rate, mate.")

Are there "clang" associations?

(6) *Irrelevance.* The patient's answer has nothing to do with the question and may not even have anything to do with the main idea being discussed. (When asked about her feelings towards her husband, the patient may answer: "Yes, it really hasn't rained much, I'm afraid my garden will be ruined.")

Are the patient's answers irrelevant?

5. Thought Content

Content of thought deals with what the patient has to say about his problems and the reason for his visit. Subtle disturbances of thought such as obsessions are not described here. It is important, however, to determine if the patient is deluded, or has suicidal thoughts or intent.

Delusions

Delusions are explanatory beliefs constructed by the patient to justify his perceptual distortions and misevaluations. These beliefs are not held by his family or community and no amount of logical reasoning can convince the patient that what he believes is not true.

Are there "wrong beliefs" (delusions)?   #

(1) *Persecutory delusions.* The patient is convinced that somebody wishes to harm him. This can be elicited by asking the patient outright if he believes somebody wishes to harm him, if he thinks he is being followed, has observed strange behaviors in people that surround him, or has felt that somebody or something is controlling his mind. An explanation for all of this should be asked of the patient.

Persecutory delusions?

(2) *Grandiose delusions.* The patient believes he is very important, may describe special powers and capacities, and may feel that he possesses a special identity. He may present himself as vastly wealthy and powerful.

Grandiose delusions?

(3) *Religious delusions.* The patient may
present a religious identity, report direct communication with God, or present himself as the
Savior or the Virgin; he may insist that he
is performing miracles, pray continuously, or
adopt a ceremonious tone of voice. Be sure to
separate fundamentalist religious beliefs
(which are normal) from bizarre religious
ideas. Note that religious delusions are
often grandiose.

Religious delusions?

(4) *Depressive delusions.* The patient may
express nihilistic thoughts, excessive guilt,
suicidal thoughts or acts, extreme hopelessness, and the conviction that "all will end,"
and "there is no tomorrow."

Depressive delusions?

(5) *Somatic delusions.* The patient has
a marked overconcern with his/her body or
bodily functions, which are described in
bizarre ways. He may state that he does not
have a heart, for example, or that he has
syphilis (despite negative laboratory results).

Somatic delusions?

Suicidal thoughts or intent

The patient should be asked about
suicidal thoughts or intent, especially if
there are signs or symptoms of depression
(no matter how mild). The question can
simply be asked, "Have things seemed so bad
that you've thought of hurting or killing
yourself?" A positive answer requires more
questions (see Chapter 10, "Suicide"), and
often a psychiatric consultation.

Is the patient suicidal?

6. Hallucinations

Hallucinations are perceptual disorders
in which the patient experiences certain
sensations without external stimuli. They
can be experienced in any sensory modality.
Differentiation should be made from illu-
sions, which are *misperceptions* that are
frequently the product of ambiguous external

Are there hallucinations?
What kind are they?

stimuli or the emotional state of the
person.

Auditory hallucinations are the most fre-   Auditory hallucinations?
quently encountered and can be explored by
asking the patient if he has heard voices
speaking to or about him which others do not
seem to hear.

Visual hallucinations should be investigated   Visual hallucinations?
by asking the patient if he sees things
that others do not seem to see.

Hallucinations of taste and odor may also be   Hallucinations of taste or
present.   smell?

Some hallucinatory experiences (for
instance, those occurring just before falling asleep) are not considered pathological;
neither are very simple hallucinations that
are not associated with other symptoms
(e.g., hearing one's name called), or those
associated with a grief reaction. Hallucinations that are visual, not particularly
bizarre, and have to do with everyday
events frequently point to an organic
brain syndrome. *Any* hallucination may
be a symptom of a nonpsychiatric organic
disorder, as may any of the signs and symptoms elicited in a mental status exam.

7. Sensorium

The patient's state of consciousness should
be determined, as well as his perception of
the environment.

(a) Orientation with regard to time,   Is the patient oriented to:
place and person. The patient should   Time? Place? Person?   #
identify the full date, the place where the
interview is occurring, and he should know
who he is as an individual within a community, not only his name. All this may be

obvious from the patient's conversation, but
if you aren't sure, *ASK*.

(b) Recent memory can be explored by
asking the patient where he lives and with
whom, when he came to the institution (if
hospitalized), or activities relating to the
current day or the day before. A
nonintrusive questions is "Who came with
you today?"

How good is recent memory?#

(c) Remote memory can be tested by
asking the patient about childhood events,
school, jobs, names of significant members
of his family, dates, and places, or simply by
noting how well he can answer questions in
the medical history.

How good is remote memory?

(d) Counting and calculation. When
evaluating this parameter, the patient's
education should be known; hasty conclusions should not be drawn concerning organicity in a person with little education.

Can the patient count and
calculate?

8. Abstract Thinking

Abstract thinking is the process by which a
person determines common characteristics
for a group of objects or situations. This
can be evaluated by asking the patient the
meaning of common proverbs. When abstract thinking is impaired, the patient may
in effect repeat the proverb, rather than
interpret its meaning.

Can the patient interpret
proverbs?

9. Judgment

This has to do with the patient's capacity
to evaluate his situation, interpret reality,
and act accordingly. Special attention should
be given to the patient's functioning at school,
at work, or within his family. The patient's
judgment, of course, is key to his following
directions given by you in a treatment plan.

Does the patient have good
judgment?   #

10. Physical Examination

The mind and body are not distinct entities. Every patient should receive some portions of a mental status exam, and every patient should have a complete physical and neurological examination. Frequently, signs and symptoms of mental illness are the most dramatic changes in the patient with an underlying nonpsychiatric organic illness; and persons with "physical" presenting complaints may have a psychiatric illness, or both a psychiatric and a nonpsychiatric illness.

Physical and neurological exam.

USE OF THIS CHAPTER

The signs elicited in the mental status examination are one key to the application of the diagnostic flow charts used throughout this book. As with signs elicited in the history, physical, or laboratory examinations, they are to be taken as only one piece of the diagnostic puzzle. Few by themselves are pathognomonic of illness in general or of a specific illness. Certain signs, however, are useful in pointing towards areas for further inquiry.

Unusual movements in the patient, if not due to a neurological disorder, can point towards a psychosis, a drug or alcohol withdrawal syndrome, or a drug or alcohol intoxication (see Chapter 7, "Organic Brain Syndromes" and Chapter 12, "Alcoholism"). Constant moving about, often accompanied by constant speech, is seen in mania (see Chapter 5, "The Syndrome of Depression"), but also in delirium (see Chapter 7, "Organic Brain Syndromes"), and also in psychosis (see Chapter 11, "Psychosis"). Antipsychotic drugs can produce profound restlessness, with pacing and inability to sit still, but not the extreme agitation seen in the above conditions.

Emotional reactions in the patient are not considered abnormal unless they are extreme or inappropriate to the situation. If the emotions are "labile" (easily brought on and/or rapidly changing), an organic brain syndrome can be considered. Extremely hostile or aggressive patients may have a paranoid psychosis (See Chapter 11, "Psychosis"). Elation or sadness should lead you to rule out an affective disorder (see Chapter 5, "The Syndrome of Depression"). An extremely blunted or highly inappropriate emotional reaction may point towards a psychosis. It is easy to overinterpret emotional reactions in patients, especially if they are highly dramatic individuals. If in doubt, a psychiatric consultation is indicated.

Thought process is perhaps the most difficult aspect of the mental status to evaluate. This is in part because of the wide variety of thought processes that can be considered normal, as well as the subtlety with which serious defects sometimes are presented. Still, some direction-finding is possible by listening for abnormalities in the thought process. A simple rule of thumb is that if you and the patient speak the same language and dialect, and yet you cannot understand much of what the patient says, a thought disorder may be present (a psychosis of a "functional" or an organic nature). In addition, if the patient generally makes sense but you perceive his answers to be irrelevant, strange, or otherwise inappropriate, consider the same conditions.

Abnormally slow or rapid thought and speech are also difficult to evaluate, unless they are severe. These signs may point towards the same conditions as do extremely slow or rapid movements.

Delusions are in general easier to evaluate than thought process and, if present, point towards a psychosis or an organic brain syndrome. In a psychosis, the delusional material often has a bizarre quality, and often is unbelievable on its face. Delusions due to organicity may sound relatively "normal," except that the clinician strongly suspects (and informants may confirm) their falsity. An example is an elderly person who believes that her family is trying to poison her. Keep in mind, however, that there is always a grain of truth in a delusion (though discovering what it is may prove difficult). In this example, the patient's family may indeed be ambivalent about continuing to care for her at home and may be considering placing her in a nursing home ("getting rid of her" in a certain sense). The patient has taken the grain of truth and has twisted it until it is scarcely recognizable. A specific kind of delusion to be aware of is that often found in a depressed person who is very concerned with his or her body and its functions. These concerns may gradually become bizarre and delusional, and this can be the first sign of a depressive psychosis (see Chapter 5, "The Synrome of Depression"). (For example, an elderly, depressed man who is overly concerned with his gastorintestinal tract may one day announce quite seriously that his bowel is "dead and rotting.")

The presence of hallucinations can point towards psychosis or organicity. As with delusions, psychotic hallucinations often have a bizarre quality, while those associated with organic brain syndromes tend to have rather ordinary content (such as seeing relatives who aren't present).

Determining whether signs from the mental status exam are of acute or insidious onset can be an important clue. For example, delusions or hallucinations of very acute onset may lead you to consider a drug or an alcohol disorder (see Chapter 7, "Organic Brain Syndromes" and Chapter 12, "Alcoholism"). Such acute onset in an elderly patient may also be drug-related (usually a side effect of a prescribed drug), or perhaps may be a sign of a cerebrovascular accident. Abnormalities in orientation, memory, and ability to caculate are, of course, cardinal signs of organic brain syndromes. The effects of drugs and alcohol are specific types of organicity to be considered. Not as well appreciated is that someone who is psychotic may appear disoriented because he cannot understand and appropriately respond to the questions asked. In this case, other signs of psychosis should accompany the disorientation (see Chapter 11, "Psychosis", and/or Chapter 5, " The Syndrome of Depression").

The patient's judgment is a key to any patient's treatment. If you fail to realize that judgment is impaired, you may give medications and instructions to the patient that he or she cannot follow.

CONCLUSION

Signs from the mental status examination should not be used to classify a patient's difficulties as "mental." Any of these signs can (and does) result from various nonpsychiatric organic illnesses. In addition, there may be a coexistence of psychiatric and nonpsychiatric organic illnesses; attempting to classify an illness as one or the other early in the evaluation may lead you astray. For further information on assessing mental functioning, see Chapter 7, "Organic Brain Syndromes."

Some clinicians are embarrassed to ask many of the mental status questions of an apparently intact patient; however, once rapport has been established, if questions about mental status are asked in the same way you ask about cardiac or respiratory symptoms, most patients will simply answer the questions with no second thought.

2.
Clinical Problems in Adults

CHAPTER 5

The Syndrome of Depression

The syndrome of depression is a very common problem encountered in general clinical practice. It is characterized by a sad mood or a pervasive loss of interest in things, associated with symptoms such as insomnia, loss of appetite, weight loss, lack of energy, feelings of worthlessness, and thoughts of death or suicide. This syndrome is one of the most frequent complaints brought to the attention of the general practitioner, whether associated with clearly established causes, isolated, or as an additional component of a medical problem. Patients, however, are likely to present vague somatic symptoms to the health professional; thus, careful interviewing is necessary to elicit specific depressive symptoms. For purposes of simplicity, in this manual the syndrome of depression will be divided into two major groups: the nonpsychotic and the psychotic depression.

CLINICAL PICTURE

Depression is found with similar features in different cultures and is characterized by periods of several weeks in which the person feels sad, unhappy, blue, uninterested in things that he/she enjoyed before; in addition, there are usually other symptoms like weight loss, lack of appetite, insomnia, lack of energy, sexual disinterest, difficulty concentrating, and suicidal thoughts or acts.

This syndrome includes a continuum of depressive disorders without psychotic features from the moderate to the very severe forms. Many times they constitute a reaction to a specific external situation (reactive or exogenous depression); at other times there is no apparent reason for the depression (endogenous depression). But since both exogenous and endogenous depression respond well to similar therapeutic approaches, no distinction is made in this volume between the two forms. If the syndrome is the response to a loss of any kind (e.g., the death of a loved person), it is called a *grief reaction*.

DIAGNOSIS

To investigate the existence of the syndrome of depression, the Syndrome of Depression Questionnaire is used. The corresponding diagnostic flow chart (Figure 5.1) is used to rule out and to identify a psychotic depression. Review of the preceding material should be an aid in case of doubt. In using the questionnaire, emphasis should be given to the *parts*. Every question is important, but item Number 1 is essential for the diagnosis of the syndrome of depression; if it is present with several items from 2 to 17, a positive diagnosis of a syndrome of depression is made. It must be remembered that symptoms caused by drugs, medicines, alcohol or illness do not count for the diagnosis of the syndrome.

SYNDROME OF DEPRESSION QUESTIONNAIRE*

	YES	NO
1. Have you had in the last month, two weeks or more during which you felt sad, blue, depressed or when you lost all interest and pleasure in things that you usually cared about or enjoyed?	—	—
2. In the last month has there been a period of two weeks or longer when you *lost your appetite*?	—	—
3. In the last month have you *lost weight* without trying to, as much as two pounds a week for several weeks?	—	—
4. In the last month have you had a period when your eating increased so much that you *gained* as much as two pounds a week for several weeks?	—	—
5. In the last month have you had a period of two weeks or more when you had *trouble falling asleep*, staying asleep, or with waking up too early?	—	—
6. In the last month have you had a period of two weeks or longer when you were *sleeping too much*?	—	—
7. In the last month has there been a period lasting two weeks or more when you *felt tired* out all the time?	—	—

*Adapted from Robins LN, Helzer JE, Croghan J, Williams JBW, Spitzer RL. NIMH Diagnostic Interview Schedule (DIS). Developed for the National Institute of Mental Health under Contract MH 278-79-0017 (DB) and Research Grant MH 33583, 1980.

	YES	NO

8. In the last month has there been a period of two weeks or more when you talked or moved *more slowly* than is normal for you? ___ ___

9. In the last month has there been a period of two weeks or more when you had to be *moving all the time*—that is, you couldn't sit still and paced up and down? ___ ___

10. In the last month has there been a period of several weeks when your *interest in sex* was a lot less than usual? ___ ___

11. In the last month has there been a period of two weeks or more when you had a lot more *trouble concentrating* than is normal for you? ___ ___

12. In the last month have you had a period of two weeks or more when your *thoughts* came more slowly than usual? ___ ___

13. In the last month has there been a period of two weeks or more when you felt *worthless, sinful, or guilty?* ___ ___

14. In the last month has there been a period of two weeks ore more when you *thought* a lot *about death*—either your own, someone else's, or death in general? ___ ___

15. In the last month has there been a period of two weeks or more when you felt like you *wanted to die?* ___ ___

16. In the last month have you felt so low you *thought of committing suicide?* ___ ___

17. In the last month have you *attempted suicide?* ___ ___

The flow chart (Figure 5.1) summarizes the diagnostic procedures the practitioner should follow once the Syndrome of Depression Questionnaire has indicated the presence of the depression syndrome and suicidal risk has been indicated. Once depressive symptoms are identified, further investigation is necessary before making a diagnosis. The role of medicines, drugs, illness, or losses should be explored as a possible basis for the symptoms. Also, findings of retardation, delusions, hallucinations, or agitation should indicate the likelihood

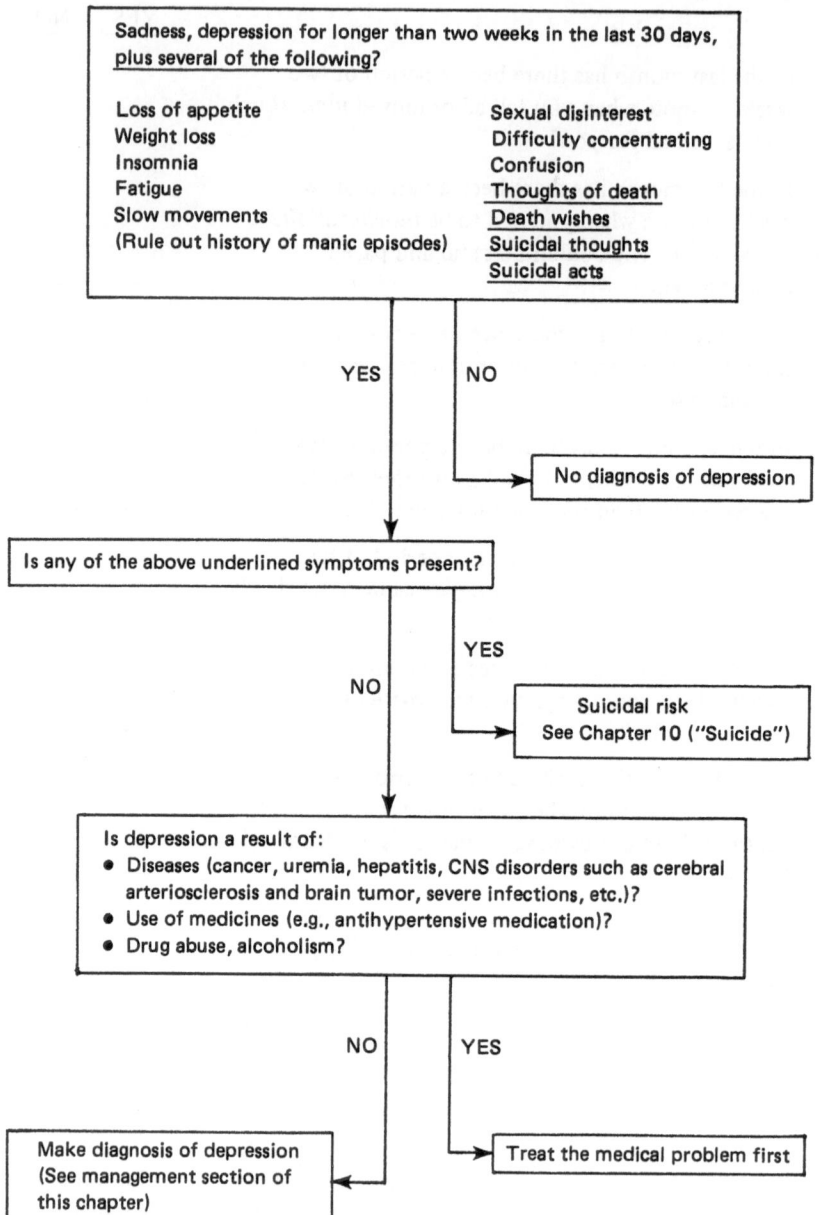

Figure 5.1 Syndrome of depression, diagnostic flow chart

of a psychotic depression, in which case a high suicidal risk should suggest careful steps regarding management. If an organic origin and psychotic elements have been ruled out, the case is diagnosed as a nonpsychotic depression.

The possibility of depression associated with medical illness, masked depression, and grief reaction should always be explored when seeing patients at the primary health care level. They will be briefly discussed below.

Depression Associated with Medical Diseases, Alcohol, or Medication

The clinician is frequently confronted with depressed patients suffering from medical diseases. Hypertensive cardiovascular disease, debilitating infectious diseases, hepatitis, uremia, and CNS (central nervous system) disorders such as arteriosclerosis or brain tumors are not infrequently associated with depression. Also, depressive symptoms can occur as a reaction to medication, alcoholism, or drug abuse. These cases should be referred for treatment of the basic problem; the depression should be considered secondary.

Masked Depression

In contrast to the above is the patient who is given repeated surgical or medical treatments without a clearly recognizable physical disorder; this patient should remind the health professional of the possibility of a masked depression. Patients with masked depression, present predominantly with physical complaints such as chronic pain (e.g., back pain, atypical facial pain, or headache); arthritic complaints; unexplained fatigue; or recurrent preoccupation with bodily complaints of a hypochondriacal nature. Depression may be present although not openly manifested; if that occurs, the administration of the Syndrome of Depression Questionnaire should help confirm the diagnosis of depression.

Grief Reaction to Bereavement

Since this is a normal response, it is important to follow just a few simple principles in dealing with grieving patients: help the person to accept the reality of the loss; suggest attendance of all relatives—especially the children—at the funeral and whatever services are held afterwards; *do not encourage prescription of sedatives*; also, do not advise people to "take a vacation" or "move to another house" since it may only encourage the denial of the loss and delay healthy grieving.

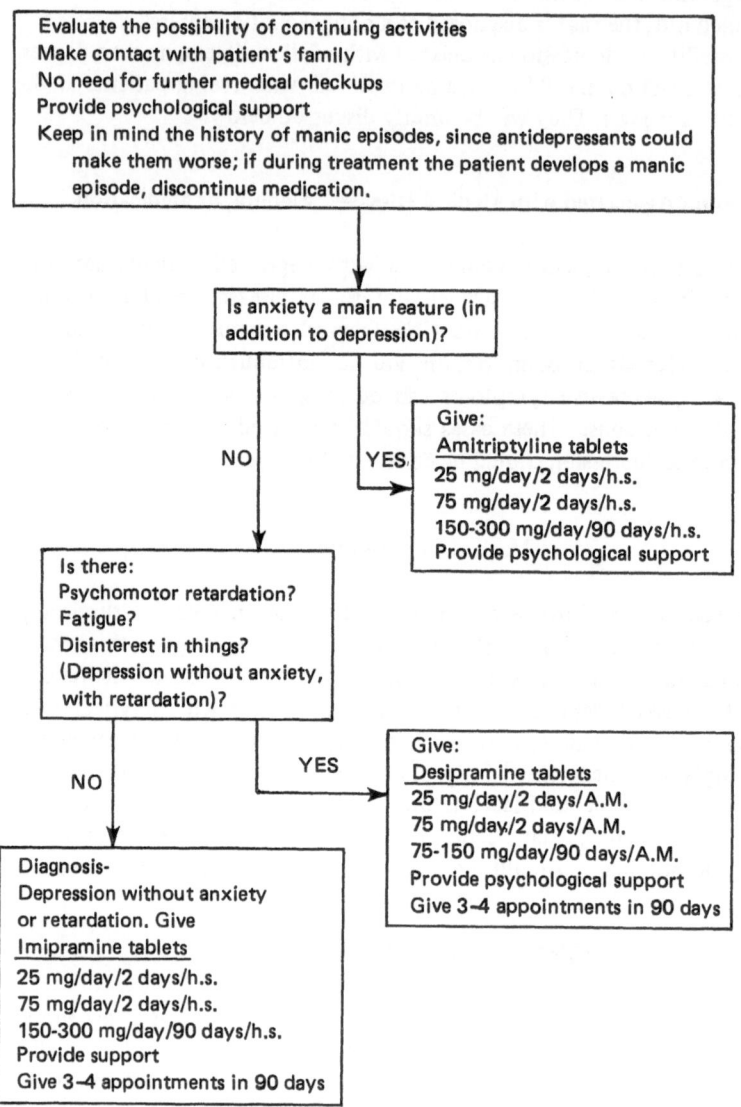

Figure 5.2 Syndrome of depression, psychopharmacological management flow chart

MANAGEMENT OF DEPRESSION

- Follow principles of clinical interviewing (see Chapter 1).
- Evaluate the possibility of the patient's continuation with routine activities (school, work, etc.).
- Allow interruption of routine activities just for a brief period if patient insists and if such a demand is congruent with the clinician's evaluation.
- Facilitate or write permission to be absent from routine activities only if appropriate.
- Explain to relatives that patient suffers an illness that can be treated and that he or she is not malingering.
- Provide the patient with support and explanations about a good prognosis if proper treatment is followed.

PSYCHOPHARMACOLOGICAL TREATMENT

The management of depression with drugs is a very effective procedure, but is generally not recommended for children. Tricyclic antidepressants are the drugs of choice and there are many of them. Three drugs will be discussed here. Being knowledgeable about them will provide the health professional with enough flexibility for a successful intervention in the pharmacological treatment of most depressions. They are amitriptyline, desipramine, and imipramine. Discussions about the use of other drugs like the MAO (monoamine oxidase) inhibitors, lithium, or CNS (central nervous system) stimulants are beyond the scope of this manual. Start with one tablet of tricyclic antidepressant the first day and ask the patient to let you know if any severe side effects occur. If that is the case, referral to a mental health specialist might be necessary. Always keep in mind that if the patient has a history of manic episodes (see Chapter 11, "Psychosis"), antidepressants could induce a manic attack.

Amitriptyline

Consider prescribing amitriptyline if *anxiety* is a predominant feature and/ or the patient suffers from insomnia, and if there is *no* psychomotor retardation. If that is the case, prescribe amitriptyline 25 mg, two tablets hs; increase by 25-50 mg per day up to 300 mg. If patient is tolerating the drug well, a faster increase in dosage is acceptable. It should be kept in mind that evident response to the treatment takes at least one or two weeks. Ask the patient to report any side effects. If there are no marked side effects and the patient shows improvement, maintain for three months. Make monthly appointments as follow-up.

The most common side effects of amitriptyline are: dry mouth, blurred vi-

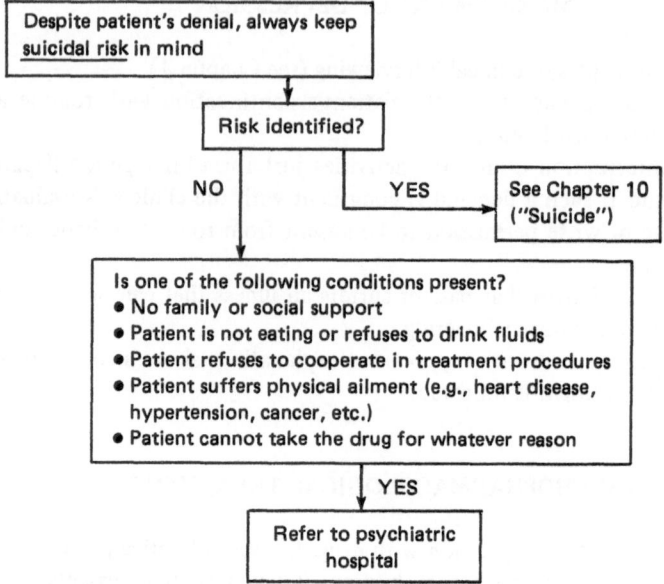

Figure 5.3 Syndrome of depression, hospitalization considerations flow chart

sion, urinary retention, and orthostatic hypotension. Be aware of specific contraindications of these drugs, especially in closed-angle glaucoma. It should be cau-
tiously used in heart disease, hypertension, and prostatic hypertropy.

Desipramine

If *psychomotor retardation* is a predominant feature (i.e., slow movements,
fatigue, lack of energy), then desipramine 25-mg tablets should be used. Start
with one tablet in the morning; after 2 days another tablet at noontime may
be added, and so on up to 75-150 mg/day. This drug can produce insomnia
if used less than eight hours before bedtime. Use for three months. Side effects
and contraindications are similar to those described for amitriptyline. This drug
is a good choice for elderly patients with depression.

Imipramine

Although slightly less sedating than amitriptyline, imipramine is similarly
effective and dosages are the same. Imipramine can also be used in place of desipramine (see Appendix I for further information).

In more severe cases of depression, the same principles and pharmacological agents are used; dosages at the upper end of the dosage range are used—up to 300 mg/day of amitriptyline or imipramine, or 150 mg/day of desipramine. In these cases the need for hospitalization needs to be carefully considered.

A picture of intense sadness, lack of energy, and psychomotor retardation with thoughts of suicide indicates a severe case of depression that requires immediate attention. If there is no response within the first week of treatment and/or the clinical picture shows some deterioration, consultation with a mental health specialist is recommended. Additional information can be found in Chapter 20, "Psychopharmacology."

By definition, a suicidal risk is high among depressed patients, despite their denial of suicidal thoughts or plans; therefore, special attention should be paid to this aspect. When there is suicidal risk, the reader should consult Chapter 10, "Suicide," for the determination of risk and for management procedures. Any of the following indications should suggest referral and/or hospitalization: (1) the absence of social or family support; (2) severity of illness; (3) the inability to take sufficient fluids and food; (4) the patient's poor cooperation; (5) a concomitant physical problem; or (6) the unwillingness or inability to take the medication, for whatever reasons. Appointments should be given 1–4 times per month, according to the progress observed; the family should be involved at all times in the follow-up; attention should be given to side effects.

REFERENCES

American Psychiatric Association. *Diagnostic and Statistical Manual of Mental Disorders, Third Edition.* Washington, D.C.: American Psychiatric Association, 1980.

Beck AT. *The Diagnosis and Management of Depression.* Philadelphia: University of Pennsylvania Press, 1973.

Paykel ES. *Handbook of Affective Disorders.* New York: Guilford Press, 1982.

Rosen H. *A Clinician's Guide to Affective Disorders.* Miami: Mnemosyne Publishing Co., 1981.

CHAPTER 6

The Syndrome of Anxiety

Anxiety can be defined as an unpleasant emotional state characterized by fear without an apparent reason or by the sensation that something uncomfortable is going to happen. Symptoms such as difficulty breathing, palpitations, dizziness, tremors, or sweating may also be present. These symptoms can occur in normal individuals under circumstances of stress. The syndrome of anxiety can be a disproportionate response to a minimal cause or can occur in the absence of a known cause. The anxiety syndrome is a common disturbance, which occurs more frequently among women than men in a ratio of 3 to 2 (Nemiah, 1975). It is seen more often in adolescents and young adults than in older adults. Anxious patients present frequently to health professionals, but they may not be identified unless anxiety symptoms are asked about specifically.

CLINICAL PICTURE

Persons suffering from chronic anxiety present one or several of the following symptoms: irritability, tension, apprehension, shyness, sensitivity to criticism of others, exaggerated worry, self-consciousness, chronic fatigue, and poor concentration. In addition, the patient may show insomnia, restlessness, and an inability to perform normal duties and responsibilities. Hostility, distrust and suspiciousness toward others are found in the more severe forms. Symptoms of depression may also be present.

DIAGNOSIS

The syndrome of anxiety as discussed in this chapter corresponds largely to the "Generalized Anxiety Disorder" as it appears in DSM-III. A positive diagnosis is made if there are symptoms in three or more of the groups assessed in the following Anxiety Questionnaire.

ANXIETY QUESTIONNAIRE

In the past month, have you experienced:

	YES	NO
1. *Motor Tension*		
Jumpy or jittery feelings or tremors of hands?	___	___
Tense or achy muscles?	___	___
Feelings of fatigue without a good reason?	___	___
Difficulty resting and relaxing?	___	___
Restlessness (inability to stand still even for one moment)?	___	___
2. *Autonomic Hyperactivity*		
Difficulties in breathing?	___	___
Hard heart beatings?	___	___
Lightheadedness?	___	___
Tingling sensations in your face, fingers, or feet?	___	___
Feelings of asphyxia?	___	___
Pain or a pressure in your chest?	___	___
Feeling that your were going to faint?	___	___
Excessive perspiration?	___	___
Sudden temperature changes (cold or hot)?	___	___
3. *Apprehension Symptoms*		
Anxious feelings without reason?	___	___
Worry without a cause?	___	___
Fear without a reason?	___	___
Pessimism in general or specifically about your own life?	___	___
4. *State of Vigilance*		
Difficulties concentrating or thinking?	___	___
Difficulties sleeping (insomnia)?	___	___
Irritability (impatience)?	___	___

The diagnosis is positive if symptoms in at least three of the four groups mentioned in the Anxiety Questionnaire have been present for one month as a minimum and if they are not due to another mental disorder, such as psychosis or depression. Even though symptoms may be found in only one or two of the four symptom groups, indicating no formal diagnosis, treatment may still need to be considered depending on the severity of the symptoms.

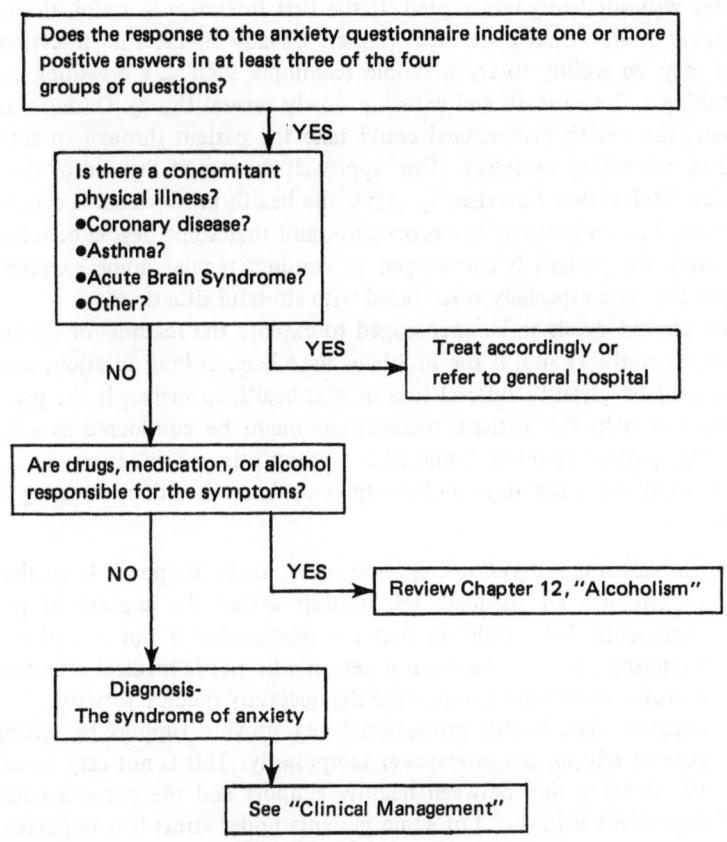

Does the response to the anxiety questionnaire indicate one or more positive answers in at least three of the four groups of questions?

YES

Is there a concomitant physical illness?
●Coronary disease?
●Asthma?
●Acute Brain Syndrome?
●Other?

NO

YES → Treat accordingly or refer to general hospital

Are drugs, medication, or alcohol responsible for the symptoms?

NO

YES → Review Chapter 12, "Alcoholism"

Diagnosis- The syndrome of anxiety

See "Clinical Management"

Figure 6.1. The syndrome of anxiety, diagnostic flow chart

CLINICAL MANAGEMENT

In the management of anxiety episodes, the first treatment procedure involves demonstrating that the present symptoms are not caused by an organic illness, but that they have a psychological basis. The implications of such recognition in the context of a primary care setting are important since no further medical checkups are necessary, assuming that medical illness has been ruled out. During the course of management, the psychological basis of anxiety should be reiterated, while recognizing that the physiological presentations are real to the patient.

The patient should be allowed to discuss thoughts regarding his or her problems without being interrupted. If the first interview is useful, the patient will appear more relaxed and feel calmer. Usually in the first interview, the patient may be willing to try a simple technique such as a breathing exercise (e.g., taking a deep breath and exhaling slowly several times). During a second interview, the health professional could take the patient through an actual rehearsal of relaxation exercises. (One approach appears at the end of the chapter under "Relaxation Exercises".) After the health professional is certain that the patient has understood the procedures and that some degree of relaxation is achieved, the patient is encouraged to conduct regular home exercises 2-3 times per day, and especially when faced with stressful situations.

The patient needs to be encouraged to explore the reasons for his anxiety (e.g., stress, conflict) and, if the problems have been of long duration, consideration should be given to referral to a mental health specialist. If the preceding steps do not help the patient, medications might be considered as a last resource. The patient could go home with a prescription of diazepam, 5 mg, once or twice a day for a few days. Follow-up in a primary health care setting should include:

1. *Emphasizing a psychotherapeutic relationship*. Emphasis is on the need to establish an adequate relationship within the context of psychotherapeutic help, insisting that the relationship is not one of a social friendship, but one between a person who needs medical attention and a professional willing to provide the necessary medical services.

2. *Support*. The health professional can provide support by letting the patient rely on the interviewer temporarily. This is not easy because of the delicate line between healthy support and the encouragement of dependent behavior. For some patients under stress it is important, for example, not to be forced (temporarily) to take any important actions. The health provider could suggest that the patient delay any major decisions until a future time. In some cases, practical suggestions regarding plans for common daily events could be discussed.

3. *Cooperation of family*. As a rule, the family should be included in the treatment plan if it is appropriate. Suggestions to relatives which are geared to minimize environmental pressures, are useful in the management of these patients.

4. *Supervision of the use of antianxiety medications*. Always insist that the patient discontinue use as soon as the symptoms improve.

5. *Subsequent meetings*. Appointments should be provided a few more times; the health provider should ensure his or her availability, particularly if the patient has experienced a panic attack.

6. *Discharge of patient*. When there is clinical improvement, the patient should be discharged and not kept under medical supervision. Subsesequent appointments are justified if symptoms reappear.

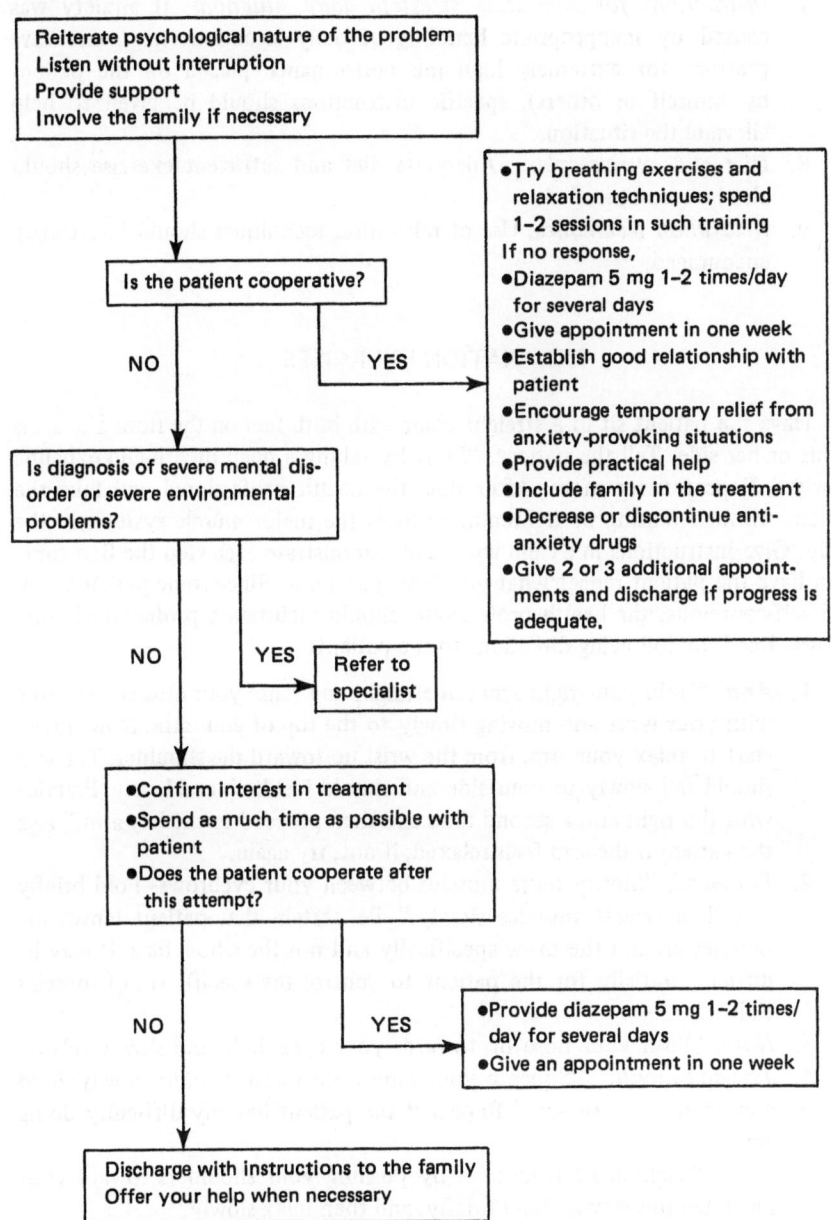

Figure 6.2. The syndrome of anxiety, management flow chart

7. *Instructions for alleviating stress in daily situations.* If anxiety was caused by inappropriate handling of daily situations (e.g., excessive pressure for extremely high job performance placed on the patient by himself or others), specific instructions should be given to help alleviate the situation.

8. *Diet and exercise plans.* Adequate diet and sufficient exercise should also be recommended.

9. *Relaxation techniques.* Use of relaxation techniques should be strongly encouraged.

RELAXATION EXERCISES

Have the patient sit in a straight chair with both feet on the floor and arms at his or her side. Tell the patient, "Start by taking a deep breath and exhaling slowly." Repeat twice more. After this, the health professional will take the patient through tensing or tightening each of the major muscle systems in the body. Give instructions in a calm voice and demonstrate each step the first time; then have the patient repeat what you have just done. Since some patients may feel self-conscious, the health professional should maintain a professional composure. Read the following directions to the patient:

1. *Arm.* "Hold your right arm out straight and tense your muscles, starting with your wrist and moving slowly to the top of your arm. Now slowly start to relax your arm, from the wrist up toward the shoulder. The arm should fall slowly to your side and should feel limp and heavy. Practice with the right arm a second time and then proceed to the left arm." Ask the patient if the arm feels relaxed; if not, try again.

2. *Forehead.* "Slowly tense muscles between your eyebrows—hold briefly and then release muscles slowly." Be certain that patient tenses the muscles around the brow specifically and not the whole face. It may be difficult initially for the patient to control the specific set of muscles called for.

3. *Nose.* "Push your nose up towards your eyes, hold and slowly relax."

4. *Jaw and mouth.* "Squeeze your mouth into a tight smile—slowly; hold and then relax—slowly." Repeat if the patient has any difficulty doing this.

5. *Neck.* "Tighten neck muscles by pushing your shoulders toward your head. Do this slowly, hold briefly, and then relax slowly."

6. *Shoulders.* "Pull your shoulders back and push them toward each other. Do this slowly, hold, and relax slowly."

7. *Stomach.* "Slowly pull stomach in, hold, and then relax stomach muscles."

8. *Buttocks*. "While continuing to sit up straight in the chair, slowly tighten buttocks, hold, and then slowly relax these muscles."
9. *Legs*. "First push right leg out so that it is parallel to the floor. Tighten muscles starting with the foot, moving to the ankle, the calf, the knee, and finally the thigh. Hold, and then slowly relax from the foot on up. Repeat the same procedure with the left leg."
10. *Whole body*. "Sit back and with eyes closed, think *RELAX*—arms, forehead, nose, jaws, neck, shoulders, stomach, buttocks, legs. Then take a deep breath and exhale slowly. Repeat."

Instruct the patient to practice these exercises several times a day, preferably when not under pressure to respond to other demands. Early morning just after rising, and just before bedtime are good times for most people. It is also possible to practice most of the relaxation exercises while riding in a car. Another important time to apply this technique is when the patient is approaching an anxiety-producing situation.

REFERENCES

Glick RA. Anxiety and related states. In: *Psychiatric Emergencies*, Glick RA, Meyerson AT, Robbins E, Talbott JA (Eds.). New York: Grune and Stratton, 1976.

Nemiah JC. Anxiety Neurosis. In: *Comprehensive Textbook of Psychiatry*, Vol. 1, 2nd Ed. Freedman AM, Kaplan HI, Sadock BJ (Eds.). Baltimore: Williams & Wilkins, 1975, p. 1199.

Pariser SF, Pinta ER, Jones BA, Young EA. Diagnosis and management of anxiety symptoms and syndromes. In: *Psychopharmacology Update*. Davis JM, Greenblatt D (Eds.). New York: Grune and Stratton, 1979.

Shader RI. *Manual of Psychiatric Therapeutics*. Boston: Little, Brown, 1975.

CHAPTER 7

Organic Brain Syndromes

An organic brain syndrome (OBS) results from a diffuse disturbance of the brain tissue function, due to any cause. The frequency of these problems within general health care is relatively high, particularly among older adults. Some of these conditions involve irreversible deterioration of brain functions; accurate identification can lead to treatment, which can in some cases prevent such deterioration. The only information included here regards differential diagnosis. No management instructions are included since the treatment of organic mental disorder should be carried out by a specialist in psychiatry or neurology.

CLINICAL PICTURE

All organic brain syndromes, independent of their cause, include disturbances of one or several of the following: memory, orientation, judgment, intellectual functions, and affect.

Memory

Immediate and recent memory disturbances and, to a lesser degree, remote memory disturbances may be present. The ability to receive and retain external stimuli may be altered. Memory retention is examined by asking the patient to repeat a series of words a few minutes after they were said; evidence of altered memory retention might be shown by failure during the immediate examination when the patient is asked to repeat the words presented earlier in the session. Remote memory is used to recall events from the past and is assessed by asking questions about general information, such as names of previous presidents of the country.

59

Orientation

Orientation is defined in three areas: time, space, and person. Examples of disturbed orientation: The patient may be unable to remember the day, the date, or the month (minor time disorientation). The patient does not know where he is (moderate disorientation as to place). The patient is unable to remember his name (major disorientation of person). An evaluation of orientation disturbance can be carried out by using the Mini Mental Status Questionnaire in this chapter.

Judgment

Judgment is a complex function, which requires the comprehension and evaluation of facts, leading to decisions that are in the best interest of the individual. The determination of whether a disturbance in judgment is present or absent is not simple and is not evaluated in the Mini Mental Status Questionnaire. Information given by a reliable informant can provide useful data. For example, some information could be obtained regarding the patient's decisions when facing difficult choices. Also, unusual actions without reasonable explanations, such as walking through dangerous streets at night, going out on a cold day without adequate clothing, or letting a stranger come into the house, are examples of poor judgment.

Intellectual Function

A fair index of intellectual function is the adequate comprehension of verbal language. Comprehension involves the capacity to follow certain instructions and to understand the logic of a given phrase. Use of some simple mathematics and testing the capacity to acquire new learning also provide ways to assess functioning. The Mini Mental Status Questionnaire is recommended to assess mental functioning. Illiteracy, educational inadequacy, and language disorders should be ruled out before using the Mini Mental Status Questionnaire. A note should be written explaining that failure in the test is not due to an organic brain syndrome, if the patient is illiterate, uneducated, or suffering from a language disorder.

Affect

There are no specific emotional responses in an organic brain syndrome. Lability, described as instability of affect, or rapidly shifting emotions, is a common feature of the organic brain syndromes (i.e., the patient laughs or cries without reason; and/or the emotional response is inappropriate, excessive, sudden or superficial).

The clinical picture may be influenced by the personality of each individual, may be aggravated by situations of emotional crisis, and/or may present during the development of a physical illness. These factors are responsible for the great variability of clinical manifestation of these syndromes.

DIAGNOSIS

The symptoms indicating a brain syndrome might be vaguely identified by a patient or relative, but many times there is no specific complaint. A more careful examination reveals some signs or symptoms that suggest "organicity." The Mini Mental Status Questionnaire can serve as a partial summary of a mental status examination. (For additional information, see Chapter 4, "The Mental Status Examination".) It should be kept in mind that the element best identified through the use of this questionnaire is the confusional state. The examination can help the clinician determine if the patient suffers an OBS, which in turn will lead to the exploration of different causes, with the corresponding clinical characteristics (see Table 7.1, Organic Brain Syndromes, Clinical Picture). Such differential is vital to the referral and further management.

MINI MENTAL STATUS QUESTIONNAIRE*

I would like to ask you some questions to check your concentration and your memory. Most of them will be easy.

	RIGHT	ERROR	REFUSAL OR CAN'T DO
1. · · · day of the month?	—	—	—
2. · · · month?	—	—	—
3. · · · year?	—	—	—
4. · · · season?	—	—	—
5. · · · day of the week?	—	—	—

---

*From Robins LN, Helzer, JE, Croughan J, Williams JBW, Spitzer RL. NIMH Diagnostic Interview Schedule. Prepared for the National Institute of Mental Health under Contract MH 278-79-0017(DB) and Research Grant MH 33583, 1980.

	RIGHT	ERROR	REFUSAL OR CAN'T DO

6. Can you tell me where we are right now?
   For instance, what State are we in?   ——   ——   ——

7. What city are we in?   ——   ——   ——

8. What are two main streets nearby?   ——   ——   ——

9. What floor of the building are we on?   ——   ——   ——

10. What is this address (or what is the name
    of this place)?   ——   ——   ——

11. I am going to name three ob-   *Apple:*   ——   ——   ——
    jects. After I have said them, I
    want you to repeat them. Re-   *Table:*   ——   ——   ——
    member what they are because
    I am going to ask you to name   *Penny:*   ——   ——   ——
    them again in a few minutes.
    Please repeat the three items
    for me. "Apple"... "Table"...
    "Penny"...
    SCORE FIRST TRY. REPEAT OBJECTS
    UNTIL ALL ARE LEARNED. (MAKE AT LEAST SEVERAL ATTEMPTS.)

12. Can you subtract 7 from 100,   RECORD:—— —— —— —— ——
    and then subtract 7 from the   (93) (86) (79) (72) (65)
    answer you get and keep sub-
    tracting 7 until I tell you to stop?   NUMBER OF ERRORS:0 1 2 3 4 5

    COUNT 1 ERROR WHEN DIFFERENCE   Can't do . . . . . . ——
    BETWEEN NUMBERS IS *NOT* 7.

13. Now I am going to spell a work   PRINT
    forwards and I want you to   LETTER:__ __ __ __ __
    spell it backwards. The word
    is WORLD, W-O-R-L-D. Spell   NUMBER OF ERRORS:0 1 2 3 4 5
    "world" backwards.

    REPEAT IF NECESSARY, BUT   Can't do . . . . . . ____
    NOT AFTER SPELLING STARTS.

		RIGHT	ERROR	REFUSAL OR CAN'T DO
14. Now what were the three objects I asked you to remember?	*Apple:*	___	___	___
	Table:	___	___	___
	Penny:	___	___	___
15. SHOW WRISTWATCH What is this called?	*Watch:*	___	___	___
16. SHOW PENCIL What is this called?	*Pencil:*	___	___	___

17. I'd like you to repeat a
    phrase after me:

    "No ifs, ands, or buts"
    ALLOW ONLY ONE TRIAL   ___   ___   ___

18. Read the words on this page
    and then do what it says.

    **GIVE PATIENT PAPER WITH
    "CLOSE YOUR EYES" PRINTED
    IN BLOCK LETTERS.**
    Code 1 if respondent closes eyes.   ___   ___   ___

19. **READ FULL STATEMENT AND *THEN*
    HAND OVER THE PAPER.**

I'm going to give you a piece of paper. When I do, take the paper in your right hand, fold the paper in half with both hands, and put the paper down on your lap.	*Right hand:*	___	___	___
	Folds:	___	___	___
	In lap:	___	___	___

DO NOT REPEAT INSTRUCTIONS OR COACH.

20. Write any complete sentence on
    that piece of paper for me.

    SENTENCE SHOULD HAVE A SUBJECT
    AND A VERB, AND MAKE SENSE.
    SPELLING AND GRAMMAR
    ERRORS ARE OKAY.   ——   ——   ——

21. Here is a drawing. Please copy the
    drawing on the same paper.

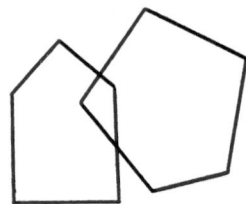

    CORRECT IF THE TWO FIVE-SIDED
    FIGURES INTERSECT TO FORM A
    FOUR-SIDED FIGURE AND IF ALL
    ANGLES IN THE FIVE-SIDED
    FIGURES ARE PRESERVED.   ——   ——   ——

SCORING INSTRUCTIONS: Count only correct responses. Score one point for
each correct answer in items 1-10, 15-18, and 20-21. Score one point for
each correct answer in items 11, 14, and 19. For items 12 and 13, use only that
item with the *most* correct answers. (For example, if item 12 has 2 errors and
item 13 has 5 errors, use only item 12 and score "3" correct responses. Highest
possible score equals 30. If the respondent scores 23 or below, cognitive impairment is implied. A score of 24-30 implies lack of cognitive impairment.

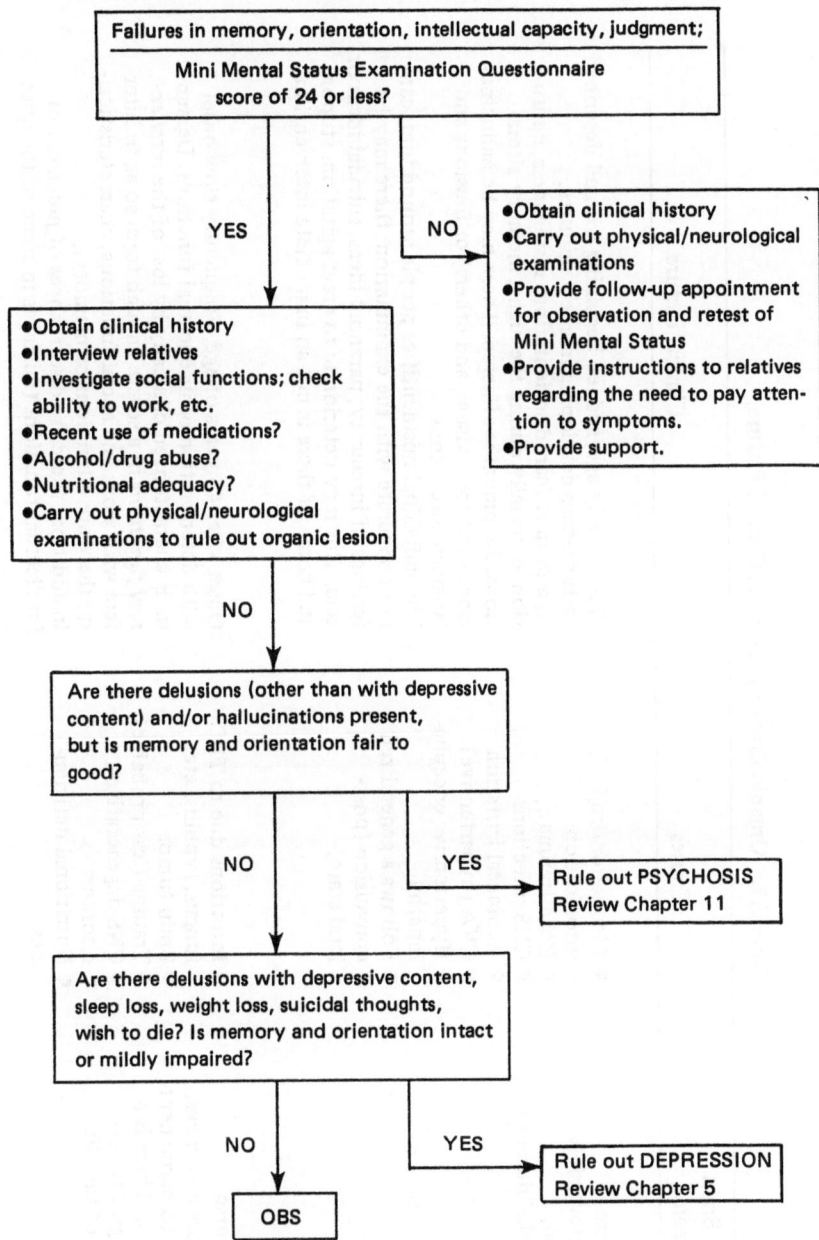

Figure 7.1 Organic brain syndromes (OBS), diagnostic flow chart

Table 7.1. Organic Brain Syndromes, Clinical Picture.

Organic Brain Syndrome	Causes	Clinical Picture
Delirium Acute course—could be irreversible if untreated; several weeks' duration	• Alcohol or drug intoxication • Head trauma • CNS infections • Meningeal irritation • CVA (hypertensive) • Hypertensive encephalopathy • Follows a generalized convulsion (postictal state)	Onset at any age; sudden beginning with all described disturbances developing in a few minutes. Symptoms: fear, disorientation, restlessness, confusion, especially during the night; memory alterations. Judgment is affected. There may be hallucinations (auditory, visual, and others) or illusions and language alterations. The individual misidentifies people around him; cannot cooperate with the examination; there may be feelings of insecurity; paranoid ideas; suicidal ideas or acts. This may deteriorate to great agitation, stupor, and coma, if there is not an immediate intervention.
Dementia Chronic course—The brain tissue damage often leads to permanent deterioration. There is a general progressive deterioration of the clinical picture.	• Infections due to TBC fungus, syphilis, etc. • Brain tumor • Trauma (less probable) • CNS degenerative disorders • Nutritional deficiencies.	Onset after 45 years of age. Frequently slow onset with deterioration of intellectual functions. Dementia is characterized clinically by loss of the *intellectual functions* in a severe enough form so as to interfere with work and social functions; characteristically, there are alterations of memory. In addition, there are disturbances of judgment or intellectual functions (mistakes in some of the ques-

Amnesic Syndrome

1. Follows: chronic alcoholism or delirium tremens.
2. Head trauma
3. Brain tumor
4. Arteriosclerosis

tions 16 to 19 of Mini Mental Status Questionnaire). *All of the above could occur in the absence of orientation disturbances.*

Generally the picture of chronic alcoholism, in addition to:
1. Gross disturbances in memory, especially in short and long-term memory.
2. Confabulation (the person creates stories to fulfill memory failures).
3. Disorientation

Drug or Alcohol Intoxication

1. Profuse and continuous ingestion of alcohol or some drugs (e.g., amphetamines)

In alcoholics, after a long period of alcoholic ingestion, if a sudden decrease in the consumption of alcohol occurs, there may be:

Does not necessarily constitute chronic alcoholism.
1. Initial period of excitation with diverse alterations in brain functions according to intoxication's severity.
2. Could last for several hours after ingestion.

1. Great anxiety; marked restlessness
2. Body tremor
3. Auditory or visual hallucinations (alcoholic hallucinosis)
4. "Grand-mal" convulsions (rare)
5. Delirium tremens (DTs). Patient appears very ill, with marked agitation; tremors; profuse perspiration; visual terrorizing hallucinations and memory disturbances.

continued

Table 7.1. Continued

Organic Brain Syndrome	Causes	Clinical Picture
Cerebral Arteriosclerosis	Predisposing factors: ● Arterial hypertension ● Genetic (family history of arteriosclerosis)	Age: Over 50 years, but frequently after age 65. Symptoms: may be initiated as a sudden state of brief confusion for which the patient suffers amnesia; or could be initiated as an epileptic convulsion. Emotional instability in the 4th or 5th decade in a person who has never suffered such symptoms. The person laughs or cries without cause; there may be a tendency toward suspiciousness, jealousy, delusional ideas, violent behavior, or confusion. The course is variable. The person forgets things easily; There are severe failures in concentration and recent memory, in contrast to an intact remote memory.
Pellagra (rare)	Nicotinic acid deficiency (B Complex)	Onset at any age. History of poor ingestion of fresh food (milk, eggs, meat, beans).

Vitamin B12 Deficiency

● Gastric surgery
● Poor diet, especially in chronic mentally ill patients.

Age: any
Depression, confusion, dementia are common among chronic mental patients

Skin symptoms: Erythema, dermatitis, skin decoloration (hands, wrists, palms, face, neck, elbows, knees). Tongue redness is characteristic. Gastric symptoms are varied and include diarrhea or constipation. CNS symptoms: Paresthesias, tremor, reflexes are diminished, convulsions are common.
Mental symptoms: Depression or dimentia, but more frequently delirium.

Folate Deficiency

Deficiency of folic acid

Age: any
Depression, confusion, dementia common among epileptics and mentally retarded, since the use of sodium diphenyl hydantoin and phenobarbital can lead to folic acid deficiency.

CLINICAL MANAGEMENT

After the clinical picture has been evaluated, a referral note to a psychiatrist or other medical specialist should summarize the more important history findings as well as the diagnostic impression. Following the specialist's evaluation, treatment and follow-up care may be referred back to the primary care professional. This will also include working with the family to help them understand the nature of the problems as well as learning how to respond to the patient's problems. The patient may require more supervision at home and, if living alone, may need the help from a visiting nurse. For some patients, referral to a rehabilitation program will be helpful in order to develop cue systems for problems such as orientation to time or short-term memory.

REFERENCES

Hendrie HC (Ed.). *Symposium on Brain Disorders: Clinical Diagnosis and Management. The Psychiatric Clinics of North America* 1978; 1(1).

Kramer JF, Cameron DC. *A Manual on Drug Dependence.* Geneva: World Health Organization, 1979.

Lazarus LW. Psychotropic Drug Management of the Organic Psychoses in the Elderly. In: *Psychopharmacology Update,* Davis JM, Greenblatt D (Eds.). New York: Grune and Stratton, 1979.

Slaby AE, Lieb J, Tancredi LR. *Handbook of Psychiatric Emergencies.* Flushing, NY: Medical Examination Publishing Co., 1975.

CHAPTER 8

The Convulsive Syndromes

The convulsive syndromes (epilepsy) originate in occasional and excessive electrical discharges in the brain. Seizure behavior involves a loss of consciousness and a wide range of other physical symptoms, which vary with the type of epilepsy.

CLINICAL PICTURE

Frequently, it is impossible to find a precise cause, but in some instances the episodes are preceded or accompanied by a variety of physical disturbances to which the convulsive syndrome could be attributed (i.e., head traumas, infections of the central nervous system, brain tumors, biochemical changes, or alcohol or drug intoxication). The disappearance of symptoms and variable intervals between convulsive episodes are typical. In many cases, a convulsive syndrome can be of brief duration; once the injury has been treated, the symptoms disappear. In other cases, the symptoms may persist unless some long-term treatment is administered. Identification and treatment of seizure disorders can result in control over seizures and minimal further consequences for most individuals.

Four different types of convulsive syndromes will be described in this manual:* Grand mal (Tonic-clonic seizures); Petit mal (absence seizures); psychomotor (focal seizures); and epileptic status.

---

*For practical reasons, a simple grouping of the most frequent categories was selected instead of the more detailed classification systems for epileptic seizures.

Grand Mal Epilepsy

The clinical picture includes a sudden onset with loss of consciousness and a fall to the floor. The body becomes rigid, followed by violent and sudden tonic and clonic movements of arms and legs. The face becomes cyanotic (purple in color). There are movements of the mouth and tongue. Other symptoms may include noisy breathing, tongue-biting, eye movements, profuse salivation, and urinary and/or fecal incontinence. This stage is followed by a period of relaxation and sound sleep; once the patient wakes up, he has no recollection of what has happened; the patient may be disoriented with respect to time or place and frequently complains of headaches, muscle aches, dizzines, and sleepiness. The crisis generally lasts from two to five minutes. Grand mal episodes can occur at any age, but are more common above the age of four and in young adulthood; in most cases the cause is unknown. This form of epilepsy responds well to the use of pharmacological agents.

Petit Mal Epilepsy

This form of epilepsy is manifested by clouding of consciousness, which usually lasts a few seconds; muscle contractures are not always present, but when they occur, are limited to movements of short muscular groups in addition to rhythmic movements of the facial muscles. The patient suddenly interrupts any activity, presents the symptoms, and returns to normality once the crisis is over. These episodes occur predominantly in children and are rarely found in patients over 20 years of age. The attacks tend to occur several times per day, frequently when the patient is under stress. They are not very frequent during exercise. This form of epilepsy is not due to a specific brain lesion.

Psychomotor Epilepsy (Temporal Lobe Epilepsy, TLE)

Psychomotor epilepsy originates in a lesion of the temporal lobe. It is characterized by loss of contact with the surrounding environment; the episode lasts 1 to 2 minutes. Onset can occur at any age. The patient does not lose consciousness or fall to the floor as in a grand mal seizure, but during the episode the patient is unable to comprehend verbal language; therefore, all attempts to communicate with the patient during the seizure are useless. The state of mental confusion lasts a few minutes after termination of the attack. One clinical feature is the psychic crisis in which a series of clinical symptoms such as sensory changes occur; the patient sees objects larger (macropsy) or smaller (micropsy) than their actual size and identifies objects further away or more brilliant than in reality. Depersonalization phenomena occur (the patient is un-

Table 8.1. Characteristics of Grand Mal Epilepsy vs. Hysteria

Grand Mal	Hysteria (Nonepileptic attack)
1. The attack occurs during the day or night; it can occur during sleep.	1. Never occurs during sleep.
2. The attack occurs both when the patient is alone and when with others.	2. Very rare when the person is alone, since secondary gain requires the presence of significant others.
3. Tongue-biting frequent.	3. No tongue-biting; only sucking movements may be observed.
4. Frequent head traumas with subsequent scars.	4. Person is careful not to be hurt; scars are infrequent.
5. Tonic-clonic movements of arms and legs.	5. Movements during the episode are disordered.
6. Urine and fecal incontinence frequent.	6. Urine or fecal incontinence very rare.
7. Loss of consciousness always present.	7. No loss of consciousness.
8. Patient does not cry during attack.	8. Patient may cry during attack.

able to recognize partially or completely his or her body); derealization occurs, (the patient is unable to recognize previously known surroundings). *Déjà vu* sensations of knowing something that he/she does now know in reality or *jamais vu*, inability to recognize something previously known, sudden episodes of fear or anxiety, auditory or visual hallucinations, and episodes of impulsive, aggressive, and violent behavior may also occur and may be very frightening to other people.

Epileptic Status

This term refers to a state of continuous or rapidly recurring seizures in which the patient does not become fully conscious between attacks.

GRAND MAL EPILEPSY

Grand Mal Epilepsy Diagnosis

The Grand Mal Epilepsy Diagnostic Questionnaire (see page 74) can help to confirm the diagnosis, but generally the differential diagnosis presents no major problems, since the clinical picture of grand mal is very characteristic. Confirmation through the electroencephalogram (EEG) is always recommended, but when it is not immediately available, treatment should be started based exclusively on the clinical findings. It should be kept in mind that the EEG frequently presents false negatives (in 30% to 40% of people with grand mal epilepsy). The differential diagnosis for nonepileptic convulsions (hysteria) is important, although hysteria is infrequently seen. The hysterical seizure has an emotional basis without a physical cause. Table 8.1 may be helpful in differentiating one from the other.

Clinical History of Grand Mal

Once the acute episode is over, all information regarding the previous history should be obtained, especially from someone who knows the patient. Past history should include information about head traumas with loss of consciousness; birth trauma, especially use of mid or high forceps; severe illnesses such as meningitis or encephalitis; toxic episodes, and use of alcohol or other drugs. It is also relevant to investigate the family history of epilepsy, headaches, and neurological disorders. Date and time of the seizure should be recorded; also, presence or absence of an "aura" indicating when a seizure is about to occur.

GRAND MAL EPILEPSY
DIAGNOSTIC QUESTIONNAIRE

Ask the following questions of patient or relatives:

	YES	NO
Has the patient suffered an attack in which he or she has fallen to the floor, with loss of consciousness and sudden movements of legs and arms?	——	——
Has the preceding occurred at the same time as one or more of the following behaviors?		
1. Contractures (spasms) of the entire body	——	——
2. Face becomes purple (cyanosis)	——	——
3. Tongue-biting	——	——
4. Profuse salivation	——	——
5. Urinary incontinence	——	——
6. Fecal incontinence	——	——
7. Attack is followed by a deep sleep	——	——

8. After sleep, the patient is unable to remember
   what happened   ——   ——
9. After sleep, the patient is confused   ——   ——
10. After the attack, the patient is dizzy and/or
    suffers headaches   ——   ——

Management of Grand Mal

A few indications are included in this chapter (see Table 8.2) about the management of convulsive disorders other than the grand mal epilepsy. Convulsive disorders are usually the responsibility of the neurologist and the patient should be referred once the diagnosis is made. However, a grand mal seizure can be easily managed at the primary health care level. The treatment objective during a Grand mal seizure is to protect the patient from possible physical injury. Furniture with sharp corners should be removed. The patient should be placed on a soft surface (bed, carpet) with a pillow under the head. To prevent tongue-biting, a tongue depressor (or other stiff object) covered by a clean cloth should be placed between the jaw, but the jaws should never be forced open. Clothing should be loose.

ANTICONVULSANT MEDICATIONS

The pharmacological treatment of convulsive disorders is generally very effective; the greatest problem is noncompliance by the patient. It is important to emphasize the need for regular daily intake of medication in order to prevent recurrence. The use of two or more anticonvulsants simultaneously is usually not recommended. A therapeutic dosage of a single medication for a trial period is usually sufficient to obtain relief. It is essential to carefully observe any side effects of different drugs for the various types of convulsive disorders (see Table 8.2). Intake of these drugs should never be interrupted suddenly. None of the anticonvulsants has curative properties; all of them reduce or eliminate the symptoms while in use. Despite this fact, the presentation to the patient should be optimistic, emphasizing that proper drug intake usually assures permanent improvement of symptoms.

Phenobarbital, an excellent anticonvulsant, is considered by many experts the drug of choice for Grand mal epilepsy. Since it is not readily available in many countries, no specific discussion is included here.

Table 8.2. The Convulsive Syndromes, Pharmacological Treatment

Type of Epilepsy	Drug Presentation	Action	Dosages (Daily)	Side Effects	Period of Treatment
Grand mal	Diphenyl hydantoin 100 mg tablets	Anti-convulsant	300 mg P.O.	Restlessness, nausea, vomiting, dizziness, skin allergy, gum hyperplasia	Indefinite
Psycho-motor (TLE)	Carbamazepine 100 mg tablets 200 mg tablets	Anti-convulsant	400/1200 mg P.O.	Drowsiness unsteadiness	Start with a low dose and continue indefinitely
Petit mal	Ethosuximide tablets 250 mg	Anti-convulsant	500/1500 mg P.O.	Drowsiness gastric irritation, skin rash, leukopenia	Indefinite
Epileptic status	Diazepam 10 mg/ampules for I. V. administration	Sedating I. V.	10 mg I. V. may be repeated in 15 minutes	Hypotension and respiratory depression	For the acute episode. If status does not stop quickly, a medical emergency exists. Continue with diphenyl-hydantoin after the episode

COUNSELING ROLE

The therapeutic contact should be long-lasting and include supportive therapy focused on helping the patient accept the disorder, crisis-intervention when necessary, environmental manipulation, and referral for family therapy if the patient and family continue to have problems with acceptance or management of this disorder. Certain restrictions on driving a car may be placed on the individual until it is clear that the medication is effective. The patient frequently needs help accepting such limitations. Other patients become so frightened of a future attack that they restrict themselves too much and need reassurance and encouragement from the health professional to resume certain functions.

REFERENCES

Gastaut H. *Dictionary of Epilepsy Definitions.* Geneva: World Health Organization, 1973.

Merritt H. *A Textbook of Neurology,* 6th Ed. Philadelphia: Lea and Febiger, 1979.

Samuels MA. *Manual of Neurologic Therapeutics.* Boston: Little, Brown, 1978.

Sutherland JM, Tait H, Eadie MJ. *Epilepsies. Modern Diagnosis and Treatment,* 2nd Ed. Edinburgh: Churchill Livingstone, 1974.

Volle FO, Heron PA. *Epilepsy and You.* Springfield, Ill.: Charles C. Thomas, 1978.

CHAPTER 9

Agitation

Agitation is a condition in which there is incessant motor activity and disordered and/or socially unacceptable behavior which occurs suddenly and/or without a specific course. An agitated state may occur in either psychotic or nonpsychotic patients. Agitation is not a disorder per se, but is symptomatic of certain clinical conditions. It is presented as a separate chapter because it is seen frequently at the primary health care level (including in hospital emergency rooms); the agitated patient usually requires emergency treatment procedures which have to be followed carefully prior to a thorough diagnostic assessment, in order to avoid injury to the patient and others.

CLINICAL PICTURE

It is useful to make the distinction between psychotic and nonpsychotic agitation. In psychotic agitation the patient appears restless and acts impulsively; arguments and fights are common and logical reasoning is not possible. The patient cannot understand what occurs around him or her and has lost touch with reality. Characteristically, he or she experiences delusions and/or hallucinations, usually of a persecutory nature. In severe cases, disorientation (of time, place, and person) and/or confusion are also present. In the above circumstances these psychotic patients constitute a high risk (dangerous behavior); therefore, their management requires fast, careful and effective procedures.

In nonpsychotic agitation, in contrast, agitation is present, but the patients do not show delusions or hallucinations; they are able to comprehend what is happening around them and remain in touch with reality. Manifestations of agitation include restlessness, impulsivity, insults, or fighting and the confrontation with logical reasoning is not accepted.

DIAGNOSIS

The application of the following Questionnaire for the Diagnosis of Agitation can facilitate the diagnostic process in case of doubt.

QUESTIONNAIRE FOR THE DIAGNOSIS OF AGITATION

In order to identify the agitated patient, at least two of the following three questions should be answered positively, of which one must be item 1. These questions would be answered from direct observation of the patient's behavior or through the interview with relatives or friends. Since both the patient and relatives or friends are under great stress, the formal and direct interview with them is rarely easy. Therefore, the following items will be verified through observation.

                                                                                     YES   NO

1. Patient appears extremely active, restless; moves
   continually from one side to the other; wrings one
   hand against the other; cries, complains, or expresses
   guilt feelings (e.g., believes himself or herself to be
   responsible for horrible acts for which he/she should
   be punished).   ___   __

2. Patient believes that other people might hurt him or her
   (delusions); hears voices that other people can't hear
   (hallucinations).   ___   __

   (NOTE: If symptoms from this question constitute the
   main clinical feature, the diagnosis would probably be
   "Acute Psychosis")

3. In addition to intense activity, patient demonstrates
   great rage; argues with belligerence for any reason and/
   or physically attacks other people.   ___   __

   (NOTE: If patient has ingested alcohol, review Chapter
   12, "Alcoholism," Differential Diagnosis section)

DIFFERENTIAL DIAGNOSIS

Rule out:

Organic Problems

The presence of an organic problem explaining the symptoms should be ruled out, e.g., CNS infections, head trauma. Special emphasis should be placed on identifying symptoms such as fever, meningeal signs, etc. If any of these problems is present, the patient should be considered a medical emergency and referred to a general hospital, with a note indicating the agitation and the detected organic problem.

Drug Abuse

Agitation or violence can be caused by the ingestion of alcohol, amphetamines, or other drugs. This possibility should always be investigated through the interview with the patient and relatives. Some physical evidence, such as an odor of alcohol, pupillary dilation (amphetamines) or eye redness (cocaine or cocabase) is helpful in making the diagnosis, but may not be present.

Seizure Disorders

Sudden episodes of unmotivated violent behavior should suggest a psychomotor epilepsy (temporal lobe epilepsy). Such episodes could be marked by a disproportionate response to some environmental factors. These situations, often clinically identical to other forms of agitation, require a different treatment; therefore precise diagnosis is essential. (See Chapter 8, "The Convulsive Syndromes.")

CLINICAL MANAGEMENT

Interviewing Principles

The principles of interviewing agitated individuals should be kept in mind. Review carefully interviewing principles, clinical history, and psychiatric examination procedures in Chapters 1-4. The interview environment should be quiet and free from other individuals, relatives, or friends. In particular, persons with whom the patient has been in conflict should not be present during the interview. It should be conducted in a quiet place in a relaxed fashion; the attitude of the interviewer should be firm but nonaggressive. It is important to try to listen without interruptions; the interviewer should be identified as an interested helper. In the case of agitated males, with a history of impulsive acts, special

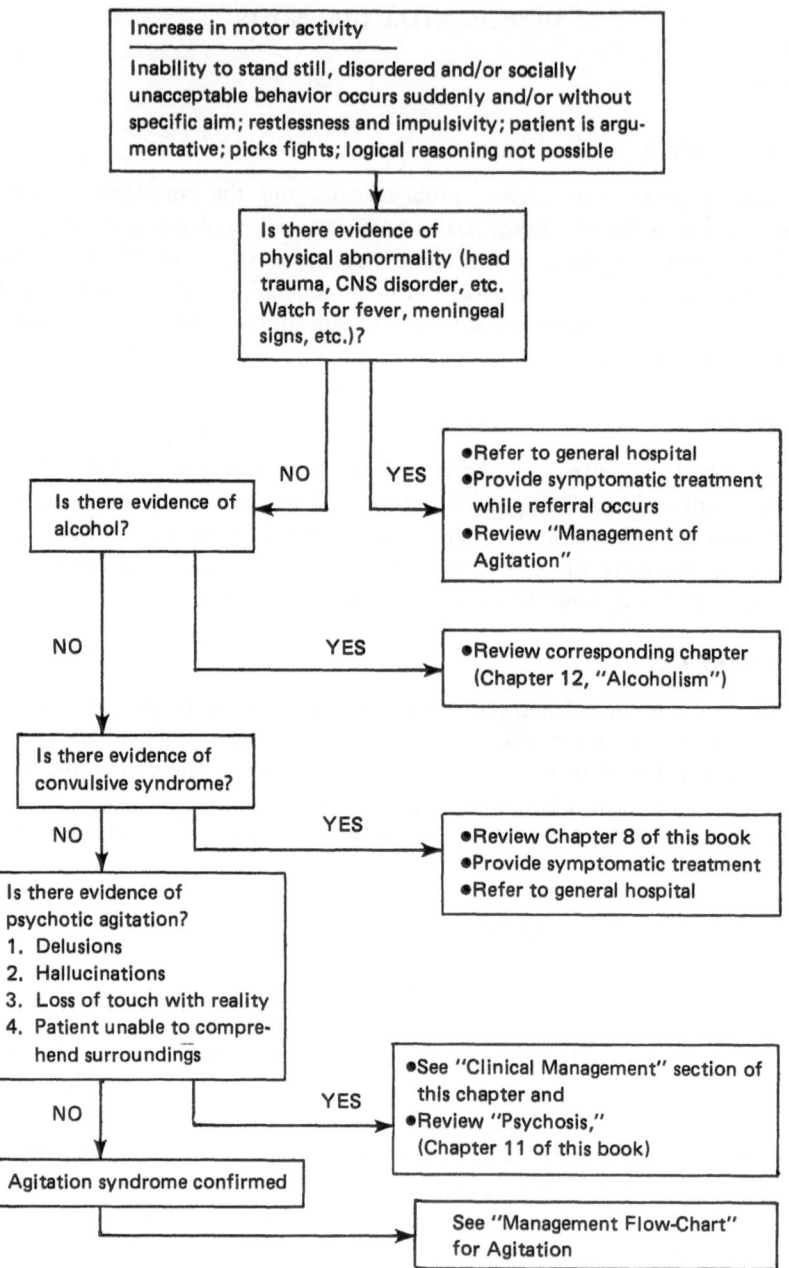

Figure 9.1 Agitation syndrome, diagnostic flow chart

care should be taken since they constitute a greater risk for violent behavior. Physical restraint is a last resort. Such procedures, although important in some circumstances, increase the patient's rage and frustration and will complicate any further therapeutic relationship.

The interviewer should never insist on pursuing the precipitating facts of the episode, since this information tends to enrage the patient. These patients are usually insecure and fragile, and a great deal of patience should be used in their management, allowing them to discuss matters of interest to them. It is essential to obtain their trust by acts of respect and interest in their situation. Also, the health professional's interest helps others to understand the importance of such attitudes toward the patient. If the above conditions are successfully provided, the chances for the patient's cooperation increase. The patient may start to talk about preoccupations, ideas, and feelings, which constitutes the cathartic beginning of the psychotherapeutic process. It is important to let the patient verbalize his rage and anxiety without focusing on details of the precipitating events. The purpose of letting the patient relate such feelings to the health professional is to help him or her calm down—not to resolve the issues presented. If necessary, complete information could be obtained at a later time, through an interview with relatives, or when the patient is calmer.

If agitation is extreme, interviewing is not indicated, and probably other measures are in order (see section on "Physical Restraint" in this chapter). It is crucial in those circumstances to have an additional trusted person available. No risks should be taken; an easy exit should always be available in an emergency or in case of a threatened physical attack on the interviewer. All dangerous instruments should be removed from the patient and his or her surroundings by appropriate personnel.

Extremely agitated people are anxious and their anxiety may be worsened by those around them who are challenging or confrontative. People should not get too close to these patients and should not provoke, threaten, or argue with, them since they are not in a position to argue logically. If the patient suggests that someone he trusts be present, this person could be called into the interview. Everybody else should be advised to stay at a distance. People should be reminded that these patients should not be mistreated, since their behavior is the result of a mental or physical disorder, which will improve when properly treated.

Administration of Drugs

Although it is likely that agitated patients will not easily accept PO medications, the first attempt should be to try haloperidol 5 mg PO or IM, repeating every half-hour up to 15-20 mg/day; this is usually sufficient. An alternative could be chlorpromazine tablets, 100 mg, up to a dosage of 300 mg per day in

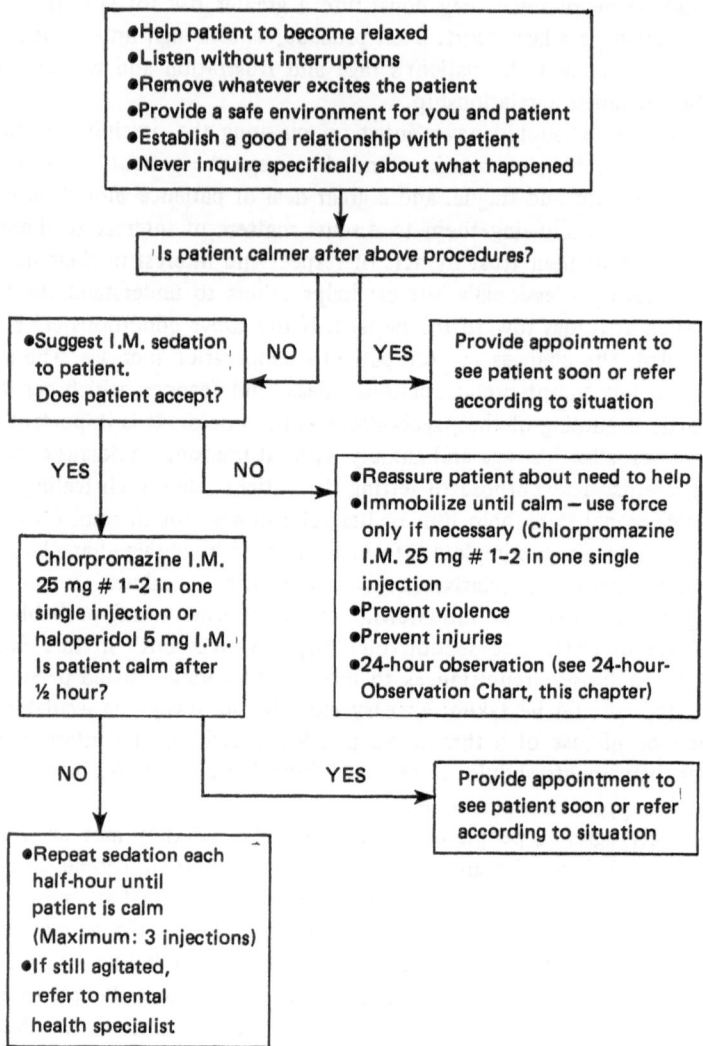

Figure 9.2 Agitation syndrome, management flow chart

one single administration. Such a dosage is usually sufficient to keep a patient calm. These drugs induce sedation and sleep. In cases of extreme agitation, immediate action is necessary through the IM administration of chlorpromazine 25 mg, one or two ampules at a time. This may have to be preceded by physical

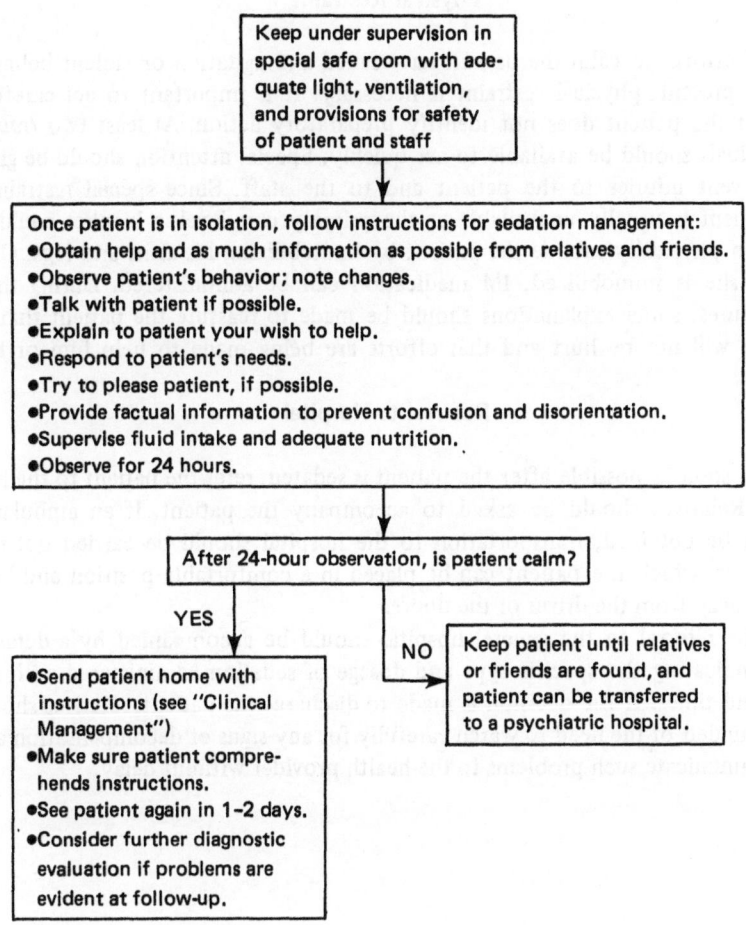

Keep under supervision in special safe room with adequate light, ventilation, and provisions for safety of patient and staff

Once patient is in isolation, follow instructions for sedation management:
- Obtain help and as much information as possible from relatives and friends.
- Observe patient's behavior; note changes.
- Talk with patient if possible.
- Explain to patient your wish to help.
- Respond to patient's needs.
- Try to please patient, if possible.
- Provide factual information to prevent confusion and disorientation.
- Supervise fluid intake and adequate nutrition.
- Observe for 24 hours.

After 24-hour observation, is patient calm?

YES

- Send patient home with instructions (see "Clinical Management")
- Make sure patient comprehends instructions.
- See patient again in 1–2 days.
- Consider further diagnostic evaluation if problems are evident at follow-up.

NO

Keep patient until relatives or friends are found, and patient can be transferred to a psychiatric hospital.

Figure 9.3. Agitation syndrome, 24-hour-observation flow chart

restraint procedures. These medications could be given every half-hour, up to a maximum of three. Restraint of the patient may be necessary in order to administer the medication. In the case of nonpsychotic, debilitated, or elderly patients, chlorpromazine should not be used; chlordiazepoxide IM 50 mg, or diazepam 20 mg IM could be used instead.

Physical Restraint

If efforts to calm the patient have failed and agitation or violent behavior is still present, physical restraint is necessary. It is important to act carefully so that the patient does not identify preparatory action. At least two *trained* individuals should be available to act quickly. Special attention should be given to prevent injuries to the patient and to the staff. Since special restraining equipment is usually unavailable at the primary care level, a blanket could be used to physically subdue the patient by immobilizing his arms and legs. Once he or she is immobilized, IM medication can be administered. During these procedures, some explanations should be made to reassure the patient that he or she will not be hurt and that efforts are being made to help him or her.

Referral to Hospital

As soon as possible after the patient is sedated, refer the patient to the hospital. Relatives should be asked to accompany the patient. If an ambulance cannot be obtained, transportation to the hospital should be carried out in a vehicle in which the patient can be placed in a comfortable position and kept safely away from the driver or the doors.

The referral to the general hospital should be accompanied by a detailed note indicating the specific type and dosage of sedation administered with the date and times. If the decision is made to discharge the patient, relatives should be reminded of the need to watch carefully for any signs of decompensation and to communicate such problems to the health provider without delay.

CHAPTER 10

Suicide

A potentially suicidal person usually thinks that life is worthless and may express a passive wish to die or to actively terminate his or her life. Suicide constitutes a complex public health problem and probably is one of the most difficult medical emergencies to prevent and handle adequately. The availability of weapons, dangerous drugs, toxic products, and poisons contributes to its frequency. Suicide is also tied to sex and age characteristics; men actually commit suicide three times as often as women, while women make three times as many attempts as men. Suicide attempts that are successful are a major problem among aging adults. Suicidal risk is increased by: physical illness, certain types of mental disorder (depression, thought disorders, alcohol and drug abuse), recent loss of a loved person, and living alone.

CLINICAL PICTURE

The most common symptoms encountered are suicidal thoughts. The patient may indicate suicidal intentions through relating that he has acquired poison, drugs, or a weapon, or may refer to a previous suicidal attempt. There are several ways in which the suicidal patient comes in contact with the health system. The family might observe strange behavior, the patient may verbalize suicidal thoughts or threats, or the patient may be referred for an unrelated medical problem during which suicidal tendencies are accidentally discovered.

DIAGNOSIS

It is important to determine if the patient suffers a depressive disorder (see Chapter 5, "The Syndrome of Depression"), since depressed patients commonly present suicidal ideation. Sadness, hopelessness, lack of sleep, guilt feelings, and other symptoms encountered in a depressive syndrome should be investigated. In addition to the patient, a relative may be asked to help complete the Depression Questionnaire (see Chapter 5). It should be kept in mind that sometimes potentially suicidal patients do not reveal these ideas in the interview; in those cases, only depressive symptoms might be cleary expressed, but the completion of the questionnaire may reveal suicidal ideas.

Once this has been done, the interview should proceed. Keep in mind the following principles: The interview provides valuable information regarding the patient and his/her circumstances; the determination of the severity of the suicidal risk is facilitated through the use of the Questionnaire (for Determination of Suicidal Risk). Complete the interview with the following questionnaire about the situations that usually aggravate the suicidal risk. These questions could be addressed to patients, relatives, or friends. One single positive response to the questionnaire, in addition to evidence of depression, suicidal ideas, or acts, constitute a moderate suicidal risk. Special attention should be given to some

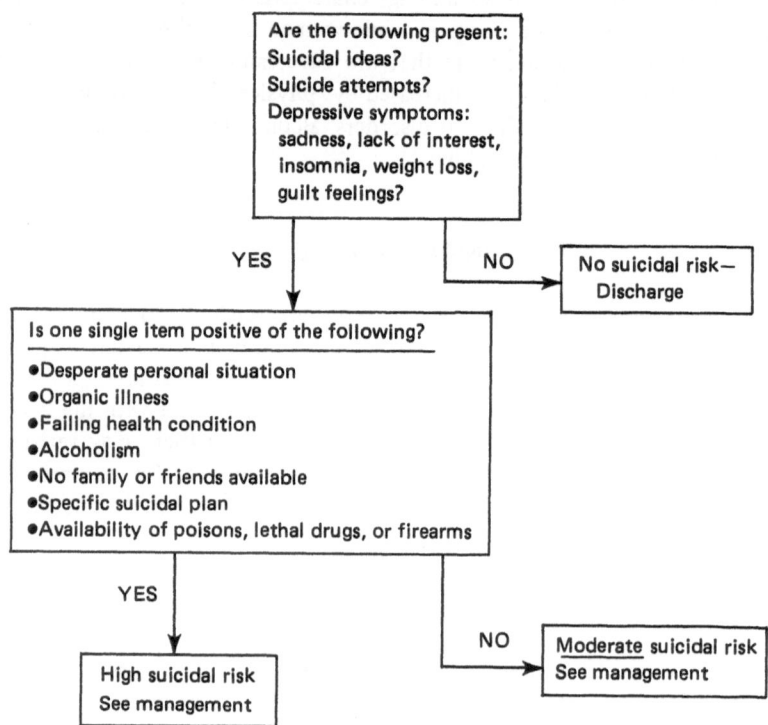

Figure 10.1.   Diagnostic flow chart, suicide risk determination

items (marked with *) since they constitute a high risk. Administer this questionnaire to persons who have indicated that they have recently thought about committing suicide or hurting themselves.

QUESTIONNAIRE FOR THE DETERMINATION OF SUICIDAL RISK

	YES	NO
1. Are you in a desperate situation of some kind (i.e., financial, legal, social, family, or other)?	—	—
2. Do you live alone?	—	—
3. Do you suffer from some severe illness at the present time?	—	—
4. Have you lost your energy to the point that everything is a tremendous effort?	—	—
5. Have you lost much weight without a good reason?	—	—
6. Have you been getting intoxicated recently?	—	—
7. Do you believe that you should be punished for something you have done?	—	—
8. Have you been hearing voices that other people cannot hear?	—	—
*9. Have you heard voices demanding that you take your life?	—	—

(Now keep in mind the answers to the Syndrome of Depression Questionnaire)

*10. You told me about some of the ideas you have regarding suicide. Have you thought about any special plan to carry out those ideas?	—	—
*11. Do you use or do you keep at home weapons of any sort like firearms, knives?	—	—
*12. Do you have access to poisons, tranquilizers, antidepressants or an excessive supply of drugs?	—	—

DIFFERENTIAL DIAGNOSIS

Drug Intoxication

Sometimes patients with suicidal ideas act under the influence of drugs or alcohol. This should be carefully assessed since treatment should address the underlying problem.

Psychosis

When the suicidal ideas are secondary to a psychosis (not an infrequent occurrence), the psychosis should be treated (see Chapter 11, "Psychosis"). The psychotic patient with suicidal ideas has a greater suicidal risk. The patient should be treated with antipsychotic medication. IM administration is preferred to acutely suicidal individuals who refuse oral medications in order to facilitate the referral to a specialized inpatient setting.

Alcoholism

Among alcoholics, suicidal ideation is common, especially when the patient is acutely intoxicated. The chances of suicide among alcoholics are greater than the average, since a depressive disorder is also frequently present in these patients. Obviously, it is important to pay attention to the suicidal problem, in addition to considering the underlying depression and alcoholism.

CLINICAL MANAGEMENT OF SUICIDE

Every patient suffering from suicidal syndrome should be considered a high suicidal risk and should receive treatment by a health professional or be referred to a psychiatric hospital according to the suicidal potential (based on seriousness of intent and other items in the Suicidal Risk Questionnaire); if adequately carried out, this constitutes an effective preventive action. If the referral to a psychiatric hospital is impossible, some management principles should be followed, keeping in mind that some symptoms are more severe than others. It is therefore important to make a distinction between the "moderate risk" and "high risk" of suicide.

The principles of interviewing and clinical history taking (Chapter 1) should be reviewed. The information regarding the details of the suicidal thought or act are important; although some people talk about suicide without carrying out the threats, they should never be taken lightly. The interviewer should talk to the patient to determine the severity of suicidal intent according to the criteria summarized through the use of the Suicidal Risk Questionnaire.

If the person is acutely intoxicated, action should be taken not only re-

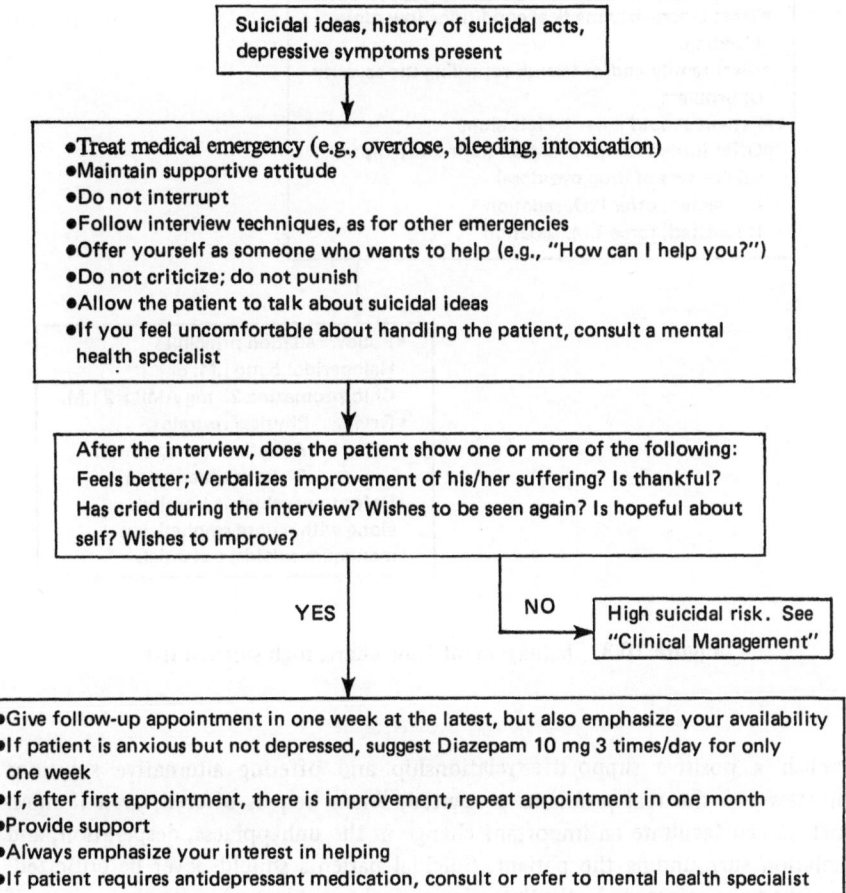

Figure 10.2. Management flow chart, moderate suicidal risk

garding the suicidal ideas but regarding the intoxication, which could be associated with violent behavior, depression, and/or sedation. If the intoxication does not improve, the patient may progress into stupor, becoming a medical emergency.

If the patient is awake, he/she should be kept in a place with good ventilation where he or she can be comfortable and can be observed continuously. In all cases, the family should be alerted as to the severity of the situation.

The patient should be listened to without criticisms, while trying to es-

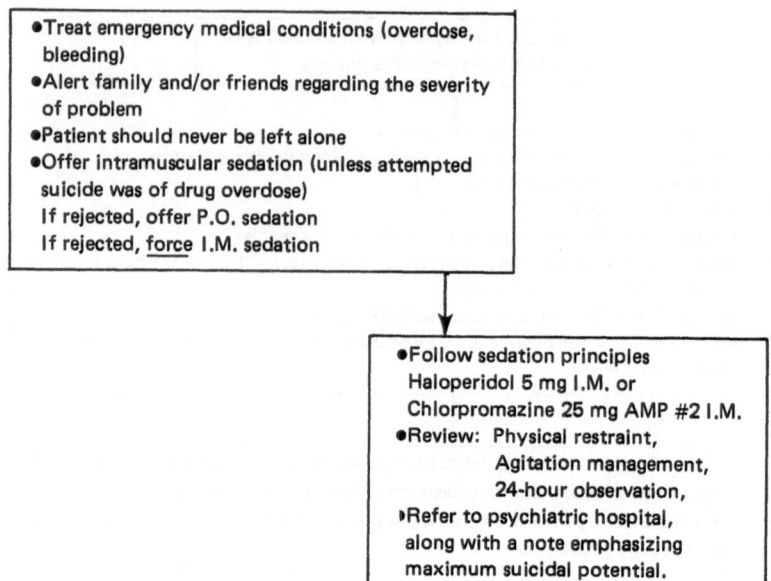

Figure 10.3.   Management flow chart, high suicidal risk

tablish a positive supportive relationship and offering alternative solutions or views to the real problems presented. When help is offered, even if minimal, it can facilitate an important change in the unhappiness, desperation, and isolation surrounding the patient. Suicidal patients should never be criticized, punished, or rejected. If the interviewer feels unable to handle the case or if the patient's behavior is considered intolerable, a different person should be asked to take care of the case.

Specific questioning about suicidal thoughts is essential since discussion about these issues frequently will help alleviate suicidal preoccupation. Some believe that discussing the suicidal thoughts with these patients might trigger a negative reaction, increasing the suicidal risk. In general, the opposite is true; suicidal patients feel relieved when they have the chance to communicate these uncomfortable thoughts without criticism. If they are able to share the "secret" with other people, they feel less guilty and isolated; they feel respected by someone willing to help. ("Someone finally understands.")

The positive aspects of the person's life should be emphasized; try to discuss with him or her those areas in which he or she is good. Try to stimulate the patient to consider getting involved in activities that he or she feels comfortable doing. This will prove to be therapeutic and should contribute to a decrease in the suicidal potential. With a patient who has either attempted suicide or who has had previous suicidal thoughts, if the interview improves the patient's spirits, the establishment of a therapeutic relationship has begun. In this situation, when it appears safe to release the patient to family or friends, asking the patient to contact the health provider when he feels suicidal can help to reinforce the patient's belief that he can cry out for help. Arrangements for contacting the clinician or an alternate health provider need to be clearly communicated. In addition, consultation with a mental health specialist, if available, is recommended.

If the patient continues to feel irritated and depressed after the interview, the suicidal risk is still high. In this case, immediate action should be taken in a decisive manner. The patient should never be left alone and all dangerous objects should be removed from his or her surroundings. An immediate referral to a psychiatric hospital (to which the patient is accompanied by relatives) is mandatory, after sedation has been given.

Sedation

Haloperidol 5 mg IM, or chlorpromazine 25 mg IM one or two, might be needed to sedate an agitated suicidal patient. (However, it should not be given in case of an attempted suicide by drug overdose.) One hour of observation after the administration of the injection should be enough to demonstrate that there is somnolence and that the patient is starting to calm down. If there is no improvement, the dosage could be repeated after one or two hours. Only when the patient shows signs of improvement is a referral safe. A specific note summarizing the information available as well as the medication given should be included in the referral report. Special emphasis should be placed on the severity of suicidal findings.

REFERENCES

Shader RI. Assessment of suicide risk. In: *Manual of Psychiatric Therapeutics*, Shader RI (Ed.). Boston: Little, Brown, 1975.
Shneidman ES, Farberow NL. *Clues to Suicide*. New York: McGraw-Hill, 1957.
Shneidman ES, Mandelkorn P. *How to Prevent Suicide*. New York:Public Affairs Committee, 1967.

CHAPTER 11

Psychosis

The term *psychosis* includes a variety of mental disorders characterized mainly by severe disturbances in thought and emotions, as well as alterations in perception and psychomotor activity not due to an organic (physical) cause. About one percent of the population suffers from psychotic disorders. Early identification and adequate management at the general health care level are crucial to prevent unnecessary human suffering. The vast majority of these patients do not receive medical attention through the most immediately accessible general medical services; contributing factors include negative attitudes of health providers towards the most severe mental disorders as well as a lack of clear guidelines regarding possible actions.

CLINICAL PICTURE

Disorders in four symptom areas will be discussed: thought; affect (emotions); motor aspects; and perceptions.

Thought Disorders

Disturbance of flow of thoughts

Disorders in the way thoughts are produced include several groups of disturbances: increased or retarded flow of thoughts; flight of ideas and blocking; absence of adequate links among associations (loosening of associations); and incoherence (what the patient expresses makes no sense).

Disturbance of content

The ideas constituting the thoughts are affected by distortion in the inter-pretation of reality; this is not modified by reasoning and it is not shared by other members of a specific cultural group. These typical manifestations of psychosis are called *delusions*. There are systematized and nonsystematized delusions. In the former, the ideas are organized and interdependent, whereas the latter are made up of independent, at times contradictory, ideas. Poor reality-testing is always present in the formation of delusions. Types of delu-sions vary according to the predominating idea (persecutory, influence, grand-eur, mystic, guilt, sin, denial, etc.). The Questionnaire for the Diagnosis of Psychosis, which follows, can help to identify some of these items.

Disorders of Affect or Emotions

Affect disturbances of psychotic individuals are diverse and present in a variety of combinations. Some of them include: lack of emotional expression, manifested by indifference towards surroundings; in an extreme form, flat affect is observed, in which all the emotional manifestations are blocked. Inap-propriate affect is the expression of an emotion that does not correspond to what the patient feels or expresses verbally (e.g., the patient laughs at the death of a loved person). The psychotic patient's emotions are withdrawn from the external world and are said to be self-invested; this may explain the interviewer's inability to "feel" or "detect" the patient's affect.

Unpredictability as well as great lability are part of the emotional mani-festations of some psychotics, who shift rapidly from happiness to sadness, from laughing to crying. Lability is found also in hysterical personalities and in people with organic brain syndromes. Ambivalence, or the coexistence of opposing emotions towards the same event, object, or person, is frequent in psychosis. Intense anxiety, usually without external precipitating factors, but occurring as a response to delusional fantasies, is also common. If anxiety takes the form of a panic attack, the patient loses control of emotions, showing disorganized motor behavior.

In major depression with psychotic features (the so-called bipolar disorder, depression, a severe form of depression not included in this manual), there are, in addition to psychotic manifestations, sadness, crying, psychomotor retardation, delusional ideas of guilt and sin, as well as suicidal ideas or acts. In contrast, increased activity, exaggerated happiness or disprotionate self-assertiveness constitute the affective components in the bipolar disorder, manic.

Motor Disorders

Motor acceleration

The psychotic person may show unusual motor activity, which in its extreme form is manic agitation. The patient talks incessantly, sings, and dances; the activity is fluctuating and purposeless. The patient does not sleep, eat, or drink, which can lead to dehydration, weight loss, exhaustion, and even death.

Motor retardation

In some patients activity is reduced to a minimum. Movement is extraordinarily slow, including gestures and verbal manifestations. An exaggerated form of this disturbance is the catatonic stupor, in which the patient does not move for hours or days, does not respond to any stimuli, and does not eat or drink. Patients in such a condition constitute a psychiatric emergency and should be referred for hospitalization.

Perceptual Disorders (Disorders in Perception)

The term *perception* is used here to describe the process of identification of stimuli arriving at the receptors of sight, hearing, taste and smell, light touch, and pain. A typical symptom of perceptual disorder is the *hallucination*, defined as a perception without an appropriate stimulus present; usually these are not differentiated from real perceptions by the individual. Auditory hallucinations (consisting of hearing voices) are the most common, while visual hallucinations are less frequently observed.

The patient is unable to recognize the idiosyncrasy of these perceptions and holds a firm belief in them. Therefore, it is useless trying to convince patients who have perceptual disorders that the hallucinations are not "real" by using logical arguments. For the psychotic individual, the hallucinations constitute reality. During the initial period of illness, hallucinations are often associated with great anxiety, the extreme of which is a panic attack; in other circumstances, especially later in the development of this illness, they can serve as comforting mechanisms for the patient, allowing adaptation to what are perceived as harsh environmental circumstances.

DIAGNOSIS

The objective identification of key psychotic symptoms is possible through the knowledge of the preceding information. The utilization of the Questionnaire for the Diagnosis of Psychosis will help recognize clinically relevant signs and symptoms.

The questionnaire has two groups of items. The first group (questions 1 to 14) constitute the basic interview. They should be asked exactly as they are written. There are two possible responses: NO, which means there is no such symptom, and YES, which means that the response is positive, after having ruled out other causes. Items 15 to 18 are not to be asked; they are to be observed during the interview.

QUESTIONNAIRE FOR THE DIAGNOSIS OF PSYCHOSIS*

In the last month (in the last 30 days):

                                                                    YES   NO

1. Have you believed people were watching you or spying on you?   ___   ___
2. Was there a time when you believed people were following you?   ___   ___
3. Have you believed that someone was plotting against you or trying to hurt you or poison you?   ___   ___
4. Have you believed that someone was reading your mind?   ___   ___

   IF YES, ASK: Did they actually know what you thought or were they just guessing from the look on your face or from knowing you for a long time?   ___   ___

5. Have you believed you could actually hear what another person was thinking, even though he was not speaking; or have you ever believed that others could hear *your* thoughts?   ___   ___
6. Have you believed that others were controlling how you moved or what you thought against your will?   ___   ___
7. Have you felt that someone or something could put strange thoughts directly into your mind or could take or steal your thoughts out of your mind?   ___   ___
8. Have you believed that you were being sent special messages through television or the radio?   ___   ___
9. Have you had the experience of seeing something or someone that others who were present could not see— that is, had a vision—when you were completely awake?   ___   ___

   IF YES, ASK: What did you see?

*From Robins LN, Helzer JE, Croughan J, Williams JBW, Spitzer RL. NIMH Diagnostic Interview Schedule. Prepared for the National Institute of Mental Health under Contract MH 278-79-0017(DB) and Research Grant MH 33583, 1980.

YES NO

10. Have you more than once had the experience of hearing
    things other people couldn't hear, such as a voice?   —— ——

    IF YES, ASK: What did you hear?

11. Did you hear voices commenting on what you were doing
    or thinking?   —— ——
12. Did you hear two or more voices talking to each other?   —— ——
13. Have you been bothered by strange smells around
    you that nobody else seemed to be able to smell,
    perhaps even odors coming from your own body?   —— ——

    IF YES, ASK: What did you smell?

14. Have you had unusual feelings inside or on your
    body—like being touched when nothing was there or
    feeling something moving inside your body?   —— ——

    IF YES, ASK: What did you feel?

(The following four items are not to be asked; they are based on observations
during the interview. A review of the text should help to answer these questions.)

15. *Thought Disorder*: Is there a verbal production that makes communication
    between two persons difficult due to a lack of comprehensible and logical
    organization (see "Thought Disorders" in text).
16. *Flat Affect*: Is there a lack of emotional response such as smile, sadness,
    irritability, etc., i.e., a total lack of facial expression? In order to write this
    as positive, it should persist during the majority of the interview (see "Dis-
    orders of Affect" in text).
17. *Neologisms*: Does the patient make use of some words without a meaning;
    does the person create new words (see "Thought Disorders" in text)?
18. *Patient appears to be Hallucinating*. Does the patient behave as if he or she
    is hearing voices or seeing things? Does the patient move the lips, but no
    words are audible? Does the patient turn the head, look over his shoulders,
    as if a voice were distracting from behind (see "Perceptual Disorders" in
    text).

    The diagnosis of psychosis is made if one or more of the symptoms referred
to are present, after it has been ruled out that they are not due to drugs, illness,
or a known physical cause, and when the symptoms have been present during
two or more weeks.

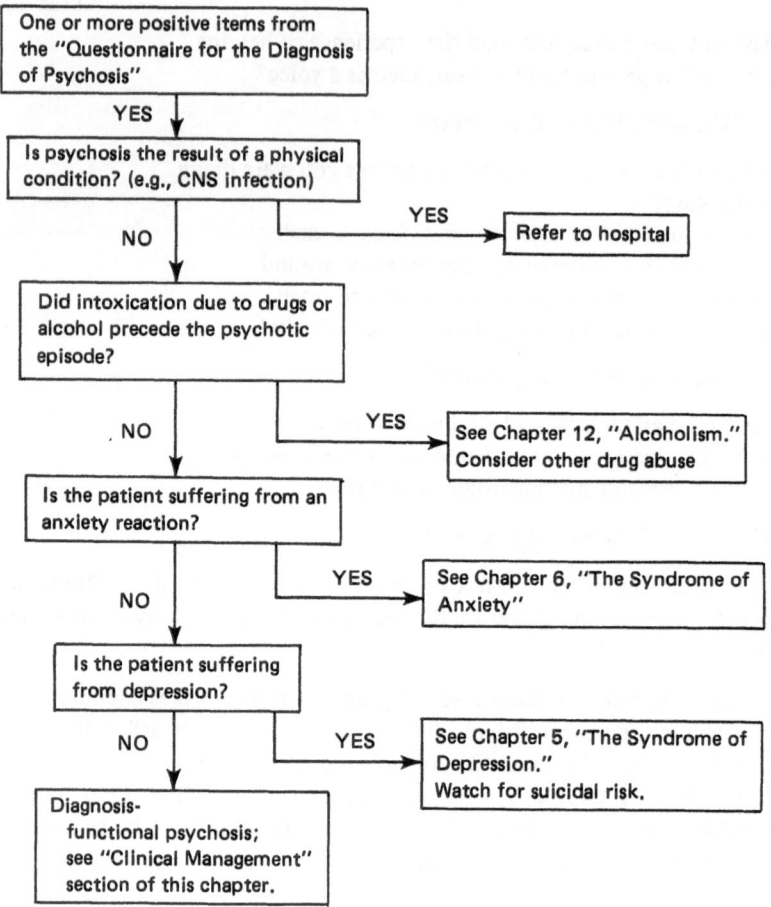

Figure 11.1.   Psychosis, differential diagnosis flow chart

DIFFERENTIAL DIAGNOSIS

First, it is important to differentiate psychosis from other organic disturbances producing psychotic symptoms (i.e., CNS infection or drug intoxication
with amphetamines, hallucinogens, alcohol, or other drugs).

Central nervous system infections

The association of psychotic symptoms and fever suggests a CNS infection. These cases should be hospitalized immediately.

Psychosis associated with drug intoxication

This constitutes an acute form of psychosis. Characteristic disturbances are found in memory and orientation. The patient appears confused and could even be disoriented as to his own person (i.e., unable to say who he or she is). Visual hallucinations or panic episodes in which the patient attempts to protect himself from "possible enemies" are not infrequent as a toxic effect of amphetamine abuse, but they can also be produced by hallucinogens or alcohol. Differential diagnosis is made by the presence of confusion, disorientation, and a history of drug or alcohol ingestion.

Psychosis vs. neurosis

The differential diagnosis between psychosis and neurosis is also of interest. Neurosis is defined as a mental disorder characterized by anxiety and/or a series of symptoms that include, among others, depression, phobias, fears, obsessions, hysteria, conversion symptoms, etc. In these disturbances:

1. There is adequate interpretation of reality.
2. The person is always able to recognize the existence of illness.
3. The social behavior of the person falls within normal limits; in neurosis the symptomatology may not be evident to other individuals, but only to the person suffering from it.
4. Emotional expression is appropriate, and is usually anxiety, restlessness, fear, depression, or a specific symptom (e.g., an obsession, phobia, etc.).
5. The inability to perform daily duties is usually not severe.
6. There are no delusional ideas.
7. There are no true hallucinations, although in some forms of hysterical neurosis, pseudo-hallucinations could be present (e.g., the person hears a voice calling his/her name).
8. Neurotic patients are well oriented in time, space, and person, except for the confusion and amnesia of a hysterical neurosis (rare).

In contrast to the above, in psychosis:

1. There is a break with reality, i.e., the person interprets reality in a distorted form according to delusions or hallucinations.
2. The person is usually unable to recognize that he or she suffers from an illness.
3. The social behavior is abnormal and quite evident to those around the individual.

4. The form of affect depends on the types of psychosis, i.e., agitation, flatness, depression, etc.
5. Social difficulties and/or inability to work are great, especially in the acute forms of the disease.
6. The form of delusional ideas depends on specifics of the delusion, i.e., guilt (depression); persecution, grandeur, suspiciousness (paranoia).
7. There are true hallucinations, for example, the patient hears insulting, threatening voices, or voices talking about him or her.
8. In the more acute phases, there is confusion and disorientation in time, space, and person.

Acute alcoholism

Frequently, acute psychotic episodes are associated with alcohol ingestion. It is difficult to determine in many circumstances if the alcohol is the cause of the psychosis or if the psychosis occurred previously and the alcohol is only an aggravating factor; therefore, it is important to determine alcohol intake and amount taken, as well as the time span of the ingestion. The final diagnosis can only be made when the person recovers from the acute alcoholic intoxication; if the psychotic symptomatology persists after the initial alcoholic phase is over, the basic diagnosis is a psychosis, to which an additional factor, alcohol intoxication, has been added.

CLINICAL MANAGEMENT

Since psychotic patients generally are extremely anxious, the first attempt should be to calm them. Instructions should be given to those caring for the patient that they are dealing with a person with an illness requiring medical treatment. These patients should be treated kindly, and their complaints should be listened to carefully without interpretation and without correcting their ideas. They should be addressed in a low tone of voice and the interview should be carried out in a private, quiet room. It is important to convey respect for their beliefs, and the interviewer should refrain from any criticism. If the patient is excited or violent, special care should be used in handling him or her (see Chapter 9, "Agitation"). Once the initial communication with the patient has been successfully established and the patient is relatively calm, some suggestions as to additional therapeutic steps could be presented.

Use of Psychopharmacological Agents

One of the most important aspects of treatment is to help the patient to calm down. In order to obtain adequate communication and better understanding of the problem, once the diagnosis has been made and drug ingestion has

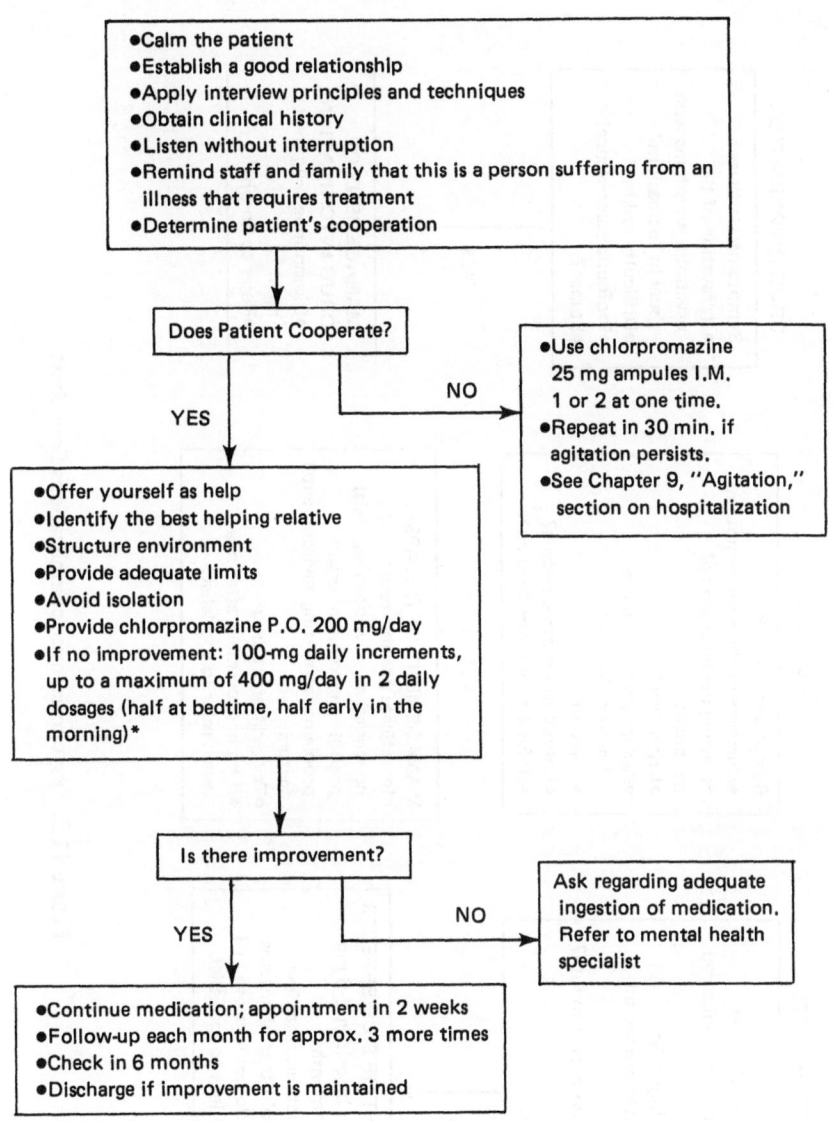

- Calm the patient
- Establish a good relationship
- Apply interview principles and techniques
- Obtain clinical history
- Listen without interruption
- Remind staff and family that this is a person suffering from an illness that requires treatment
- Determine patient's cooperation

Does Patient Cooperate?

YES

NO

- Use chlorpromazine 25 mg ampules I.M. 1 or 2 at one time.
- Repeat in 30 min. if agitation persists.
- See Chapter 9, "Agitation," section on hospitalization

- Offer yourself as help
- Identify the best helping relative
- Structure environment
- Provide adequate limits
- Avoid isolation
- Provide chlorpromazine P.O. 200 mg/day
- If no improvement: 100-mg daily increments, up to a maximum of 400 mg/day in 2 daily dosages (half at bedtime, half early in the morning)*

Is there improvement?

YES

NO

Ask regarding adequate ingestion of medication. Refer to mental health specialist

- Continue medication; appointment in 2 weeks
- Follow-up each month for approx. 3 more times
- Check in 6 months
- Discharge if improvement is maintained

*NOTE: If not certain of regular ingestion of the drug (if you suspect or know of patient noncompliance), administer fluphenazine decanoate 25 mg ampules I.M.

Figure 11.2. Psychosis, management flow chart

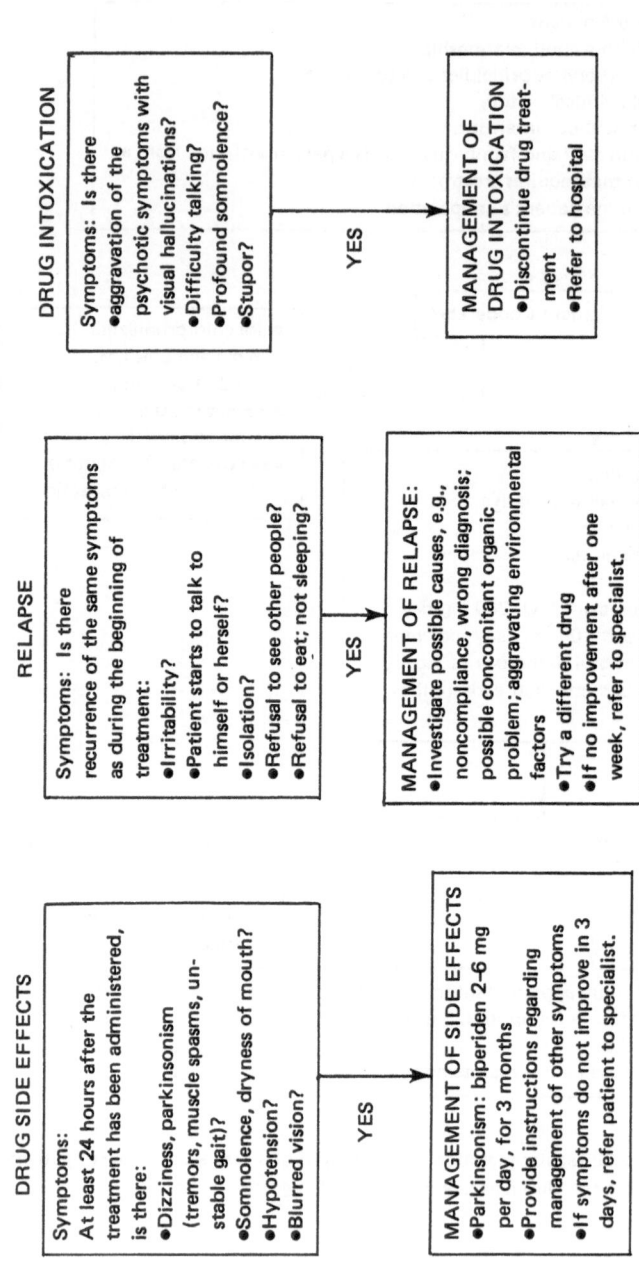

Figure 11.3. Psychosis, drug complications flow chart

DRUG SIDE EFFECTS

Symptoms:
At least 24 hours after the treatment has been administered, is there:
●Dizziness, parkinsonism (tremors, muscle spasms, unstable gait)?
●Somnolence, dryness of mouth?
●Hypotension?
●Blurred vision?

YES

MANAGEMENT OF SIDE EFFECTS
●Parkinsonism: biperiden 2-6 mg per day, for 3 months
●Provide instructions regarding management of other symptoms
●If symptoms do not improve in 3 days, refer patient to specialist.

RELAPSE

Symptoms: Is there recurrence of the same symptoms as during the beginning of treatment:
●Irritability?
●Patient starts to talk to himself or herself?
●Isolation?
●Refusal to see other people?
●Refusal to eat; not sleeping?

YES

MANAGEMENT OF RELAPSE:
●Investigate possible causes, e.g., noncompliance, wrong diagnosis; possible concomitant organic problem; aggravating environmental factors
●Try a different drug
●If no improvement after one week, refer to specialist.

DRUG INTOXICATION

Symptoms: Is there
●aggravation of the psychotic symptoms with visual hallucinations?
●Difficulty talking?
●Profound somnolence?
●Stupor?

YES

MANAGEMENT OF DRUG INTOXICATION
●Discontinue drug treatment
●Refer to hospital

been ruled out, the early use of psychoactive drugs is essential. Chlorpromazine is an excellent medication for acute psychotic episodes, especially if one or several of the following features are present: agitation, hallucinations, delusional ideas, severe anxiety, restlessness, fear, suspiciousness, and/or violent behavior.

In agitated psychotic patients, it is usually necessary to initiate with 200 mg a day of chlorpromazine for the first 24 hours. If the patient's symptoms continue or if the patient is unable to sleep, progressive increments of 100 mg per day, up to a maximum of 400 mg/day, divided in two dosages (half at bedtime, half early in the morning) are indicated.

If this dosage is not sufficient, the patient should be referred to a mental health specialist, because higher dosages are associated more frequently with secondary effects and complications. In cases of severe agitation, chlorpromazine IM is indicated to obtain faster relief of symptoms, 25 mg chlorpromazine ampules, one or two at a time, constitutes an adequate dosage for an emergency situation. If the patient is still agitated and has not improved after the first half-hour, half the dosage may be repeated (see Chapter 9, "Agitation"). For maintenance purposes, in unreliable patients, fluphenazine decanoate 25 mg ampules, IM, is an excellent alternative (see Appendix, "Psychopharmacology").

Duration

In general, it is important to maintain the drug as long as it is necessary to keep symptoms under control. One to three months of treatment should be tried before discontinuation. Improvement should be judged not solely on the absence of symptoms, but on adequate performance in the interpersonal, social, academic, and work areas. The measurement of such an ill-defined term as *improvement* is difficult, but it should take into consideration the patient's status prior to the present episode as a parameter. If improvement is not obtained after a few days, referral to a mental health specialist is necessary.

Precautions

The most common secondary effects are: orthostatic hypotension, somnolence, and dryness of the mouth. In general, side effects are more intense at the beginning of treatment, decreasing as treatment goes on. If side effects are very intense, a gradual reduction of the dosage to a minimum is advised. Hypotension, characterized by dizziness or fainting, could be ameliorated by having the patient lie down.

Chlorpromazine and fluphenazine are generally safe drugs; nevertheless, due to their hypotensive effects, they are not recommended in old or debilitated individuals.

Other side effects include tremor of hands and fingers, muscle spasticity, excessive salivation, and unstable gait; these are among the most common symptoms of parkinsonism, a disorder that occurs in about 10% of patients receiving these drugs. The treatment is antiparkinsonian medication, such as 2 to 6 mg biperiden per day, for approximately 4 to 8 weeks or as long as necessary. Another alternative is Trihexiphenidil HCl, 2 to 6 mg per day (used as for biperiden). In some patients, side effects of antipsychotic drugs can be so bothersome that other drugs should be tried, such as thioridazine (see Appendix, "Psychophamacology").

Environmental Intervention

In addition to the psychopharmacological treatment, psychotherapeutic principles should be used. These include improving the patient's communication with other people in the environment and raising his or her low self-esteem. Contact with healthy and cooperative individuals is beneficial, since such actions will permit the patient to assimilate adequate socialization skills.

The patient's surroundings should be structured without being excessively restrictive, since the latter will increase anxiety. The organization of specific programs to be carried out by the patient to completion, with easily measurable outcomes, will help improve his or her self-esteem. Isolation should be avoided; psychotic patients should be treated in their own home environment as soon as the acute phase ends.

Management of Psychotic Patients by the Family

Although the involvement of family members usually refers to patients with the chronic forms of psychosis, the basic principles apply equally well to patients with acute psychosis. It is essential that the family participate actively in the handling of the psychotic patient; relatives should be informed regarding the nature of the patient's illness and regarding desirable attitudes for the family to adopt (i.e., nonpunitive, nonargumentative). The name of the drug the patient is receiving, the place where medication can be easily obtained, the number of tablets the patient should be taking daily, the precise dosage, how long the medication should be taken, and possible problems caused by using the drug (side effects) need to be communicated clearly to the family. Although this may sound simple, information is surprisingly absent in many circumstances. The cost of treatment should be estimated to help the family facilitate adding this expense to the family budget. It is important to emphasize that the patient's improvement should not be expected as soon as treatment begins, but that it will take several weeks. At least one person in the family should be identified as more closely related to the patient's management and should supervise the pharmacological treatment. Any changes suggested in the treatment should be related to this person in addition to relating them to the patient; this key person should also inform health providers about the appearance of difficulties during treatment.

Noncompliance

Noncompliance is the most common cause of treatment failure with psychotic patients. It is essential to ascertain that the patient is taking the prescribed drug; several questions should be asked of the patient and of the key relative (i.e., the number of tablets purchased, number of tablets utilized, number of remaining tablets in the bottle), as this information allows objective conclusions regarding medication intake. It is also necessary to check with the patient and relatives about socialization activities, since they are a key aspect in the rehabilitation.

Follow-up

The follow-up appointments should be scheduled every 2–4 weeks, according to the needs of the particular patient. The patient's progress should be assessed in the following areas: modification of symptoms, secondary effects of drugs, quality of social interactions, daily activities, interpersonal relationships, initiative in starting new tasks, interest in work, and ability to get involved in leisure activities.

Changes in the patient's symptoms can be examined through the questionnaire for the Diagnosis of Psychosis (in this chapter), with confirmation obtained from relatives regarding these facts. The suitability of the medication can further be indicated by the presence or absence of drug side effects. If there is improvement, the same treatment could continue; if not, an attempt should be made to determine the reasons for treatment failure by consulting a mental health specialist.

REFERENCES

Paykel ES. *Handbook of Affective Disorders*. New York: Guilford Press, 1982.

Perry S. Acute psychotic states. In: *Psychiatric Emergencies*, Glick RA, Meyerson AT, Robbins E, Talbott JA (Eds.). New York: Grune and Stratton, 1976.

Rosen H. *A Clinician's Guide to Affective Disorders*. Miami: Mnemosyne Publishing Co., 1981.

Shader RI. *Manual of Psychiatric Therapeutics*. Boston: Little, Brown, 1975.

Snyder SH. *Biological Aspects of Mental Disorder*. New York: Oxford University Press, 1980.

CHAPTER 12

Alcoholism

An alcoholic has been defined by the World Health Organization as any person whose consumption of alcohol goes beyond the traditional and customary "dietary" use, or the ordinary compliance with the social drinking customs of the whole community concerned. Alcoholism is a chronic illness with certain identifiable characteristics, including progressive impairment of physical, emotional, and occupational functioning as a direct result of alcohol use. It is a progressive problem with frequent relapses, which seldom gets medical attention in the early stages.

CLINICAL PICTURE

The clinical picture is characterized by chronic, excessive, and persistent ingestion of alcohol, to the point of dependence, tolerance, and withdrawal symptoms. The alcoholic, when confronted with the excessive ingestion of alcohol, as a rule denies the problem.

Psychological dependence refers to the need to use a drug repeatedly without consideration of the consequences; when it is accompanied by physical symptoms, it is called *physical dependence. Tolerance* refers to the need for progressive increments of alcohol to obtain the same initial effect. Withdrawal symptoms appear after excessive ingestion of alcohol is terminated. The alcoholic usually provides innumerable explanations about the reasons for the alcohol ingestion; usually the alcoholic's explanations tend to minimize the problem to himself and to others. The need to drink makes him very able to create the proper circumstances to drink (happy occasions, sad ones, or no occasions at all). It is not uncommon for the alcoholic to seek friends among whom the excessive use of alcohol is well accepted. In such circumstances, social sanctions for drinking exist; after all, the alcoholic can say that his or her behavior is not different from what everyone else does. What ultimately happens is that alcohol dependence that has gone unnoticed leads to drinking alone, irritability when sober, restlessness, and arguments about petty, unimportant matters. This may progress to verbal or even physical aggression.

Very frequently, alcoholics present depressive symptoms; some authors believe that alcoholism is a masked form of depression. Also, a variety of organic symptoms such as gastritis, thoracic pains, palpitations, and headaches, may be reported. The alcoholic may use drinking as a treatment for uncomfortable feelings and bothersome symptoms. Temporary relief only serves to reinforce the need to use alcohol further; unfortunately, this relief is not long-lasting, and the consequences of increased dependence are more serious.

The patient may also start to experience memory failures or blackouts during periods of alcohol ingestion; during the blackouts, the alcoholic may carry out risky or complicated acts (driving long distances, committing socially unacceptable acts, fighting, etc.). Some of these behaviors can also occur in normal individuals while they are acutely intoxicated; nevertheless, in alcoholic patients such behaviors are a strong indicator of deterioration. In more advanced stages, the patient who continues excessive drinking shows further social, work, and family deterioration, along with the most severe organic consequences, such as liver damage. Withdrawal symptoms start to appear at this point; they may also be seen at an earlier stage.

Social and Family Disturbances

Chronic alcoholism is associated with a reduction in social activities. The patient reduces work-related social contacts, work satisfaction, performance, and efficiency. Obvious financial consequences frequently occur. Marital conflicts terminating in broken marriages are common. Often, chronic alcoholism is associated with automobile accidents, street fights, and problems with the law.

Organic Disturbances

There is deterioration in physical functioning. There are increased intellectual difficulties, especially in memory and attention. Gastritis, gastric ulcer, and liver disorders preceding cirrhosis are the reasons that most commonly bring alcoholics in contact with the medical profession. It is not therefore the alcohol abuse per se, but the most serious medical consequences that force these individuals to consult the health professional. The health professional needs to be in a position to make an accurate diagnosis, confront the patient in a kind but forceful manner—perhaps for the first time—with the illness, and discuss the severity of the consequences and the need for treatment.

Acute Alcohol Intoxication

The patient who has been drinking excessively for several hours appears drunk; behavioral disturbances are evident, and there is no response (or a negative response) to external attempts to modify such behavior. People with acute alcohol intoxication lack control of their behavior, which may become provocative and aggressive. They are prone to irresponsible, obscene, or dangerous acts. The patient appears disoriented in time, space, and/or person, and can be confused or unable to follow simple instructions. There is lack of motor coordination and also a disturbance in the equilibrium, along with rapidly changing emotional states.

Alcoholic Stupor

Alcoholic stupor is an extreme form of alcoholic intoxication preceded by the symptoms of acute intoxication. After excessive alcohol ingestion, agitation develops, followed by stupor in which the patient only responds to pain stimuli. The patient appears asleep, the face is red, breathing is noisy and accompanied by a strong alcohol odor. Questions need to be asked in a loud voice; however, if the patient is semicomatose, he or she will not respond. When this is so, the patient's serum ethanol level should be tested.

Withdrawal Symptoms

Withdrawal symptoms usually occur in chronic alcoholism (continuous consumption for several years), once drinking is abruptly discontinued or substantially decreased.

Tremors

Tremors of the entire body, especially of the extremities, constitute the mild form of withdrawal symptoms. These movements can occur alone or can be associated with other symptoms after discontinuation of or decrease in alcohol intake. No convulsions or loss of consciousness is present. The clinical examination does not necessarily reveal an alcohol odor.

Alcoholic hallucinosis

This situation usually occurs 1 to 3 days after discontinuation of alcohol consumption. Therefore, an alcohol odor should not be expected; the patient is oriented; the typical clinical picture is one of auditory and visual hallucinations with intense anxiety to the degree of panic; delusional persecutory ideas are frequently associated with agitation. These patients are of acute danger to themselves and should be put on suicide precautions.

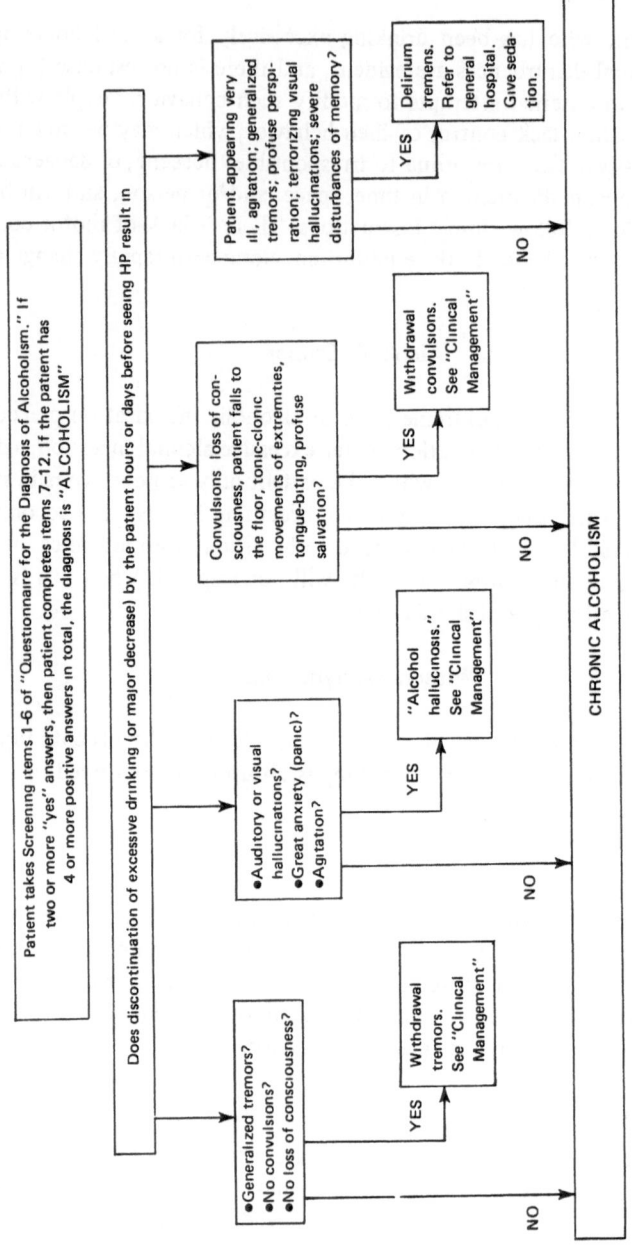

(Patient or relatives or friends mention alcohol as a problem.
The patient probably consults primarily for a medical problem.)

Patient takes Screening items 1-6 of "Questionnaire for the Diagnosis of Alcoholism." If two or more "yes" answers, then patient completes items 7-12. If the patient has 4 or more positive answers in total, the diagnosis is "ALCOHOLISM"

Does discontinuation of excessive drinking (or major decrease) by the patient hours or days before seeing HP result in

• Generalized tremors?
• No convulsions?
• No loss of consciousness?

YES → Withdrawal tremors. See "Clinical Management"

NO

• Auditory or visual hallucinations?
• Great anxiety (panic)?
• Agitation?

YES → "Alcohol hallucinosis." See "Clinical Management"

NO

Convulsions loss of consciousness, patient falls to the floor, tonic-clonic movements of extremities, tongue-biting, profuse salivation?

YES → Withdrawal convulsions. See "Clinical Management"

NO

Patient appearing very ill, agitation; generalized tremors; profuse perspiration; terrorizing visual hallucinations; severe disturbances of memory?

YES → Delirium tremens. Refer to general hospital. Give sedation.

NO

CHRONIC ALCOHOLISM

Rule out other mental disorders, i.e., depression, psychosis, anxiety, etc.
Rule out other physical symptoms, i e., diabetes, gastric ulcer, liver deficiency, etc

IF OTHER PROBLEMS ARE RULED OUT, SEE "CLINICAL MANAGEMENT" FOR SECTION ON TREATMENT OF CHRONIC ALCOHOLISM.

Figure 12.1. Alcoholism, diagnostic flow chart

Delirium tremens

The patient appears very ill, confused, and disoriented. He or she is likely to experience memory failures, marked agitation, body tremors, profuse sweating, and visual hallucinations (frequently of small insects) that can provoke a state of panic. This profound anxiety state makes an interview impossible and constitutes a medical emergency that should be handled in a general hospital. The coexistence of a physical illness is not rare and frequently precipitates and aggravates the delirium tremens.

Convulsions

Alcohol withdrawal convulsions may occur 24 hours after discontinuation of drinking, although convulsive episodes 2 to 3 days after withdrawal are not uncommon phenomena. When convulsions occur in chronic alcoholism, the clinical features are identical to grand mal seizure (see Chapter 8, "The Convulsive Syndromes"), which include loss of consciousness; a fall to the ground, body spasms, mainly of arms and legs; tongue-biting; and profuse salivation.

DIFFERENTIAL DIAGNOSIS

The differential diagnosis usually presents no difficulty, although the clinical picture can be confounded since drug abuse or other mental disorders can occur simultaneously. However, when alcohol withdrawal symptoms are mild, the diagnosis of alcoholism may be missed entirely and symptoms may be seen as having an organic basis.

Drug Abuse

It is relatively common to find alcoholism occurring in combination with abuse of some other psychoactive agent, since alcoholics seek relief of discomfort and symptoms by whatever they find useful (i.e., sedatives or hypnotics). This constitutes a multiple addiction.

Concomitant Mental Disorders

A depressive disorder is commonly associated with alcoholism. If the depressive symptoms preceded the alcohol problem, the diagnosis will most likely be depressive disorder and the alcoholism can be considered a secondary situation. Other mental disorders that can precede or coexist with alcoholism are psychosis, anxiety reactions, and different types of personality disorders, all of which require specific management considerations.

QUESTIONNAIRE FOR THE DIAGNOSIS OF ALCOHOLISM*

(Screening items 1–6)

"You mentioned some circumstances in which alcohol appears to be a problem. . ."

                                                                                    YES NO

During the last month:
1. Have you sometimes thought that you were drinking
   too much?   ___ ___
2. Have you been told by your family, friends, or your
   priest/pastor that you are drinking too much?   ___ ___
3. Have you had academic or work difficulties or lost a job
   due to drinking (i.e., work or school absences)?   ___ ___
4. Have you been drinking consistently for two or more
   days?   ___ ___
5. Sometimes, when the amount of drinking decreases or
   when you stop drinking, have you had tremors, "attacks," convulsions, delirium tremens, or have you
   heard voices or have you been seeing things that other
   people couldn't see or hear?   ___ ___
6. Have you had liver problems, jaundice, pancreatitis,
   stomach problems, blood vomiting, tingling of the feet,
   or difficulties with your memory when you were not
   drinking?   ___ ___

If two or more of the above items are answered "yes," complete items 7–12.

7. In order to control their drinking, some people
   promise themselves not to drink before 5 p.m.
   or never to drink alone. Has that occurred to you?   ___ ___
8. Have you needed a drink as you woke up (before
   breakfast)?   ___ ___
9. Have you had difficulties driving a vehicle due to
   drinking, or have you had accidents, or have you
   been arrested for being drunk?   ___ ___
10. Have you been arrested due to drinking or for
   bothering people while drunk?   ___ ___

*Adapted from Robins LN, Helzer, JE, Croughan J, Williams JBW, Spitzer, RL. NIMH Diagnostic Interview Schedule. Prepared for the National Institute of Mental Health under Contract MH 278-79-0017(DB) and Research Grant MH 33583, 1980.

11. Have you had fights while drunk?   —— ——
12. Have you had blackouts as a consequence of
    drinking; that is, have you been drinking so much
    that the following day you couldn't remember what
    you did or said?   —— ——

(If there are four or more positive responses in the total questionnaire, make a diagnosis of alcoholism.)

CLINICAL MANAGEMENT

Acute Alcoholic Intoxication

Due to the self-limiting nature of this disturbance, initial management can be restricted to clinical observations until recovery. Family members should be instructed to watch for withdrawal symptoms or a change in the state of consciousness (i.e., stupor). As a rule, sedation is not recommended. If necessary, (e.g., if the patient shows withdrawal symptoms and/or agitation, but not stupor), give diazepam IM 10 mg ampules, 1 or 2 times in 24 hours. If the patient is agitated, review Chapter 9 of this book.

During an acute episode, breathing should be facilitated; any possible obstacles should be removed such as dental prosthesis or mucus. If the patient is asleep, the head should be turned on one side in order to prevent bronchial aspiration. Vital signs should be checked frequently; any deterioration constitutes a reason for hospitalization. After the acute episode, irritability and insomnia (mild withdrawal symptoms) can be managed through the use of diazepam tablets 5 mg, 1-2 per day for a maximum of one week.

Stupor Associated with Alcoholic Intoxication

The same principles mentioned previously as for intoxication are applied, except for sedation. No sedation is used, since sedation can precipitate a comatose state.

Tremors

This is one of the manifestations of alcohol withdrawal that can disappear spontaneously, but careful observation is recommended, since tremors can deteriorate into a more severe clinical picture.

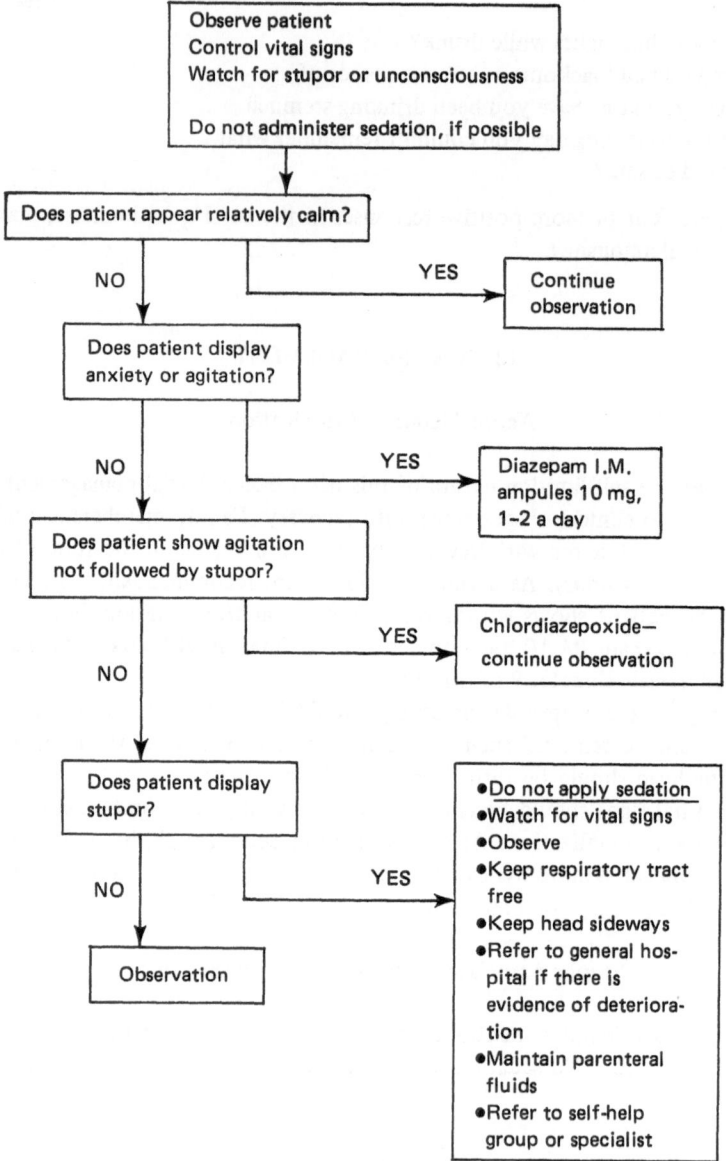

Figure 12.2. Alcoholic intoxication, management flow chart

Alcoholic Hallucinosis

Hospitalization is the procedure of choice; until that is possible, close observation and minimal stimulation are important; the interviewer should ask simple questions regarding family, hobbies, or anything that the patient could enjoy talking about. This can take the patient's attention away from delusional or hallucinatory preoccupations. The patient suffering from alcoholic hallucinosis might require heavier sedation; IM chlordiazepoxide could be used.

Convulsions

Similar management principles apply to alcoholic convulsions as to other convulsive syndromes, with the major exception being that *anticonvulsants are not prescribed*.

Delirium Tremens

After sedation, these patients should be referred to a general hosptial. Chlordiazepoxide 25 mg ampules, 50-100 mg IM, every 4 to 6 hours until the patient is calm, are recommended for sedation purposes. Most patients suffering withdrawal from alcohol suffer concomitant nutritional disorders and vitamin deficiencies (especially of thiamine), problems that should be considered as a priority for medical treatment.

General Recommendations

The following initial management principles apply to withdrawal from alcohol at any stage:

1. Apply interview principles; review agitation management principles (see Chapter 9);
2. Listen attentively; do not interrupt or criticize;
3. Review history of alcohol consumption with patient (also with family and friends), including situations and conditions under which drinking occurs;
4. Try to keep patient oriented to the immediate environment;
5. Keep patient in a quiet, well-lighted, and relaxed environment; people should not crowd around the patient;
6. Give thiamine 100-200 mg, IM, 3 times per day; also folic acid 1-5 mg daily, or multivitamins.

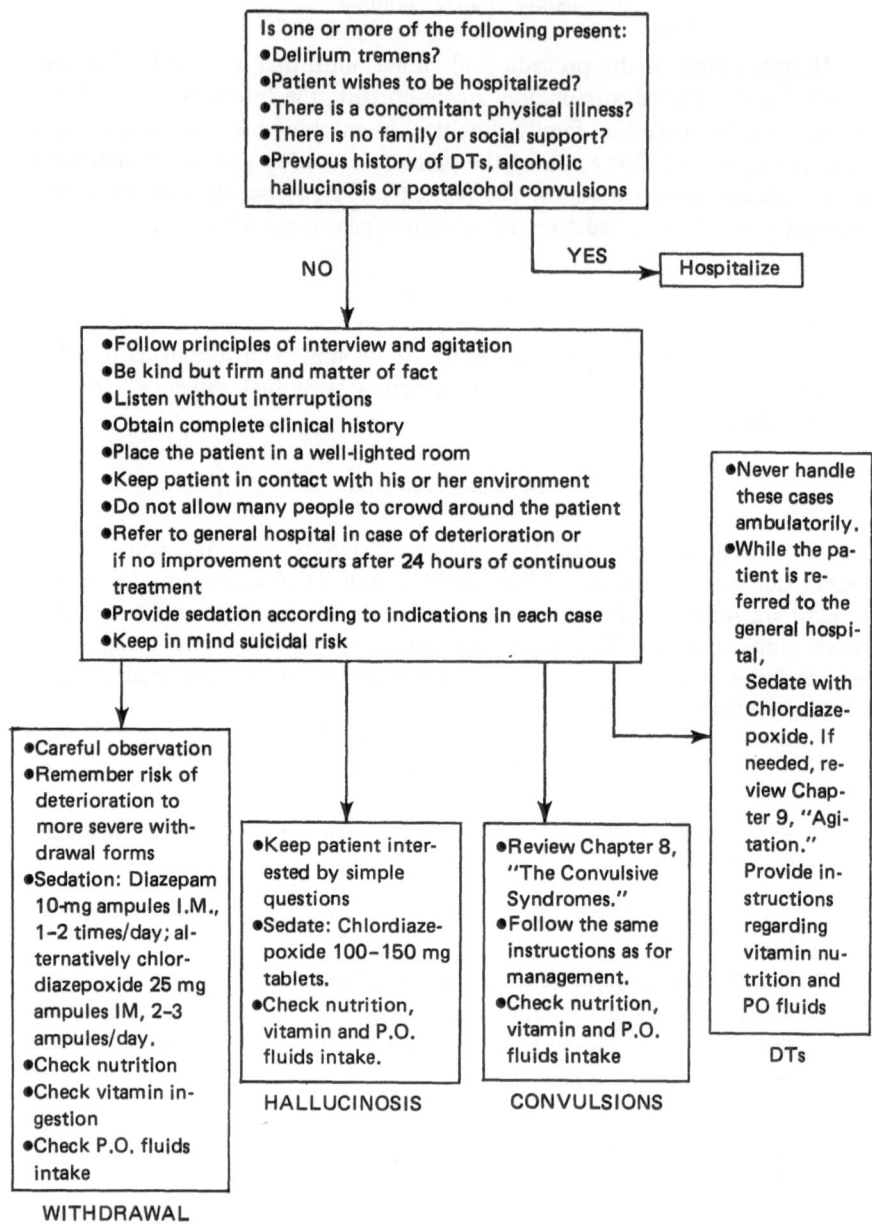

Figure 12.3. Flow chart, withdrawal syndrome management, alcoholism

Considerations Regarding Hospitalization

Delirium tremens always constitutes a medical emergency and invariably requires referral to a general hospital or a center for alcohol detoxification. Other withdrawal states may or may not require hospitalization, according to the severity and/or specific circumstances; some of these include:

1. Request by patient to be hospitalized because he or she considers it to be a serious problem, or because the patient is afraid he or she will continue drinking.
2. Coexistence of a physical illness, e.g., diabetes, hypotension, heart disease, liver disorder;
3. Lack of adequate family or social support;
4. Previous history of alcoholic hallucinosis or delirium tremens.

Further steps in the withdrawal protocol depend upon whether the patient is treated on an inpatient or outpatient basis.

Inpatient Management

1. Chlordiazepoxide 50 mg stat (PO or IM), and 50 mg every hour until the patient is calm.
2. Give up to 400-600 mg chlordiazepoxide (total dose) to the point of somnolence.
3. Every day reduce drug dose 25%, up to 200 mg daily (proceed more slowly if the patient gets hypotensive, hypertensive, etc, but not if he only has the "shakes").
4. Do not prescribe a "maintenance" dose of chlordiazepoxide. Change to disulfiran (Antabuse), or to a definitive treatment plan for other mental conditions (e.g., tricyclics, if depression is also diagnosed). Also, get patient concurrently involved in AA (Alcoholics Anonymous) or another type of long-term treatment.

Outpatient Management

1. Chlordiazepoxide 50 mg stat (PO or IM), and 50 mg every hour until the patient is calm.
2. Give up to 400-600 mg chlordiazepoxide (total dose) to the point of somnolence.
3. *Only* give 1 day's worth of medication at a time, and *only* to a sober friend or family member. (Give several capsules to a family member to give to the patient if he or she is really shaky, but if the extra pill is used for 2 days consecutively, hospitalize to at least get treatment

going.) One danger is that the patient may attempt to manipulate the family member into giving additional medication.

4. If there is alcohol on the patient's breath on a return visit, or if a friend or relative reports that the patient has been drinking, discontinue medication and hospitalize. Tell the patient on the first day that you will hospitalize him or her if he or she resumes alcohol consumption.

5. The dosage of chlordiazepoxide can be withdrawn more slowly than with inpatient management but dosage should be decreased at least 10% a day;

6. Do not prescribe "maintenance" medication. Instead, get patient involved with longer-term treatment, such as AA.

Chronic Alcoholism

Chronic alcoholism is a frustrating condition to treat, because the patient has frequent relapses; the objective of treatment is not definitive care, but, instead, keeping the patient sober. Self-help groups like Alcoholic Anonymous (AA) are one of the most effective sources for referral of chronic alcoholics. AA is usually not medication-oriented, while some other alcoholic-helping agencies are. The health professional's role is that of a caring professional who attempts to recommend the best help for the patient, while also helping the patient to accept the treatment plan. For example, in the process of referring the patient to AA, putting the patient into contact with an AA member known to the health professional may help to reduce the patient's fears and doubts about using such help. The patient is not likely to follow through until he or she wants to stop drinking. Thus, multiple approaches to the patient may be needed before a successful referral is made.

When an outpatient approach such as AA is not successful, specialized institutional settings to rehabilitate alcoholics should be considered. The length of stay is normally close to one month, during which various educational and therapeutic approaches are directed intensively toward the alcoholic's drinking behavior as well as toward his or her life goals and personal situation.

REFERENCES

Alcoholics Anonymous. New York: Alcoholics Anonymous World Services, 1955.
Fajardo R. *Helping Your Alcoholic Before He or She Hits Bottom.* New York: Crown Publishers, 1976.
Fort J. *Alcohol: Our Biggest Drug Problem.* New York: McGraw-Hill, 1973.
Mendelson JH, Mello NK. *The Diagnosis and Treatment of Alcoholism.* New York: McGraw-Hill, 1979.

Rada RR, Kellner R. Drug treatment in alcoholism. In: *Psychopharmacology Update*, Davis JM, Greenblatt D (Eds.). New York: Grune and Stratton, 1979.

Steiner C. *Games Alcoholics Play*. New York: Grove Press, 1971.

3.
Clinical Problems in Children

CHAPTER 13

Psychological Problems and Psychiatric Disorders of Childhood and Adolescence: An Overview

This chapter and the subsequent ones address psychological problems and psychiatric disorders specific to childhood and adolescence. Chapter 13 covers life crises and psychological problems, preceded by some general discussion of assessment and clinical management techniques. The psychiatric disorders presented in the subsequent chapters are: hyperactivity (attention deficit disorder); developmental disorders of childhood (specific learning disabilities); conduct disorders; anxiety disorders; disorders with physical symptoms (enuresis, encopresis, and stuttering); and mental retardation. These disorders were selected based on the frequency of occurrence in a child population, the strong likelihood of presentation to a health professional, and the possibility of some intervention at the primary health care level.

Certain rare disorders such as childhood autism (seen in about 3 out of 10,000 children) are not presented in this manual. A number of conditions described in the preceding chapters on adult disorders are also found in children and adolescents. When the diagnostic criteria and treatment are similar for children and adults, the reader should refer back to the appropriate preceding chapter. Some psychiatric conditions described in this manual may be found in both children and adults (see Table 13.1).

Initial considerations relevant to working with childhood disorders follow the same basic principles as with adults, as outlined in Section 1 of this book. These include the steps required to establish a relationship and interviewing techniques. Establishing the relationship requires the ability to create trust between the health professional and the patient(s) (parent and child). Communicating warmth, concern, and acceptance of the patient and his or her problems

125

Table 13.1.   Psychiatric Conditions and
                       Age of Onset

Condition	Possible Age of Onset
Alcoholism	Late childhood; adolescence more likely
Depression	From infancy on
Epilepsy	From birth on
Psychosis	Adolescence
Suicide	Pre-adolescence to Adolescence

represent the basic ingredients. The first session is normally not sufficient to allow the patient to open up fully about behavioral or emotional problems; several sessions for critical assessment of such problems should be anticipated.

Interviewing Techniques

Interviewing techniques can be carefully selected to facilitate the development of a trusting relationship and to obtain the information necessary to assess a problem. These include:

- Establishing eye contact
- Listening carefully without interrupting
- Reflecting on feelings: "As I understand what you are telling me, you are concerned about . . ."; or "When you are alone you feel afraid."
- Making clarifying statements: "Based on what you've told me, you are most concerned about . . ."
- Using open-ended questions initially: "How do you feel about Johnny's behavior?" followed later by more specific probes.
- Use of noncommittal responses or silence: statements like "hum, uh, huh, oh," or silence provide encouragement to the child or parent to further describe a problem, thoughts, or feelings and to allow time to organize a response.
- Providing reassurance, when the problem has been sufficiently assessed to do so: "The great majority of children who wet their beds at age 5 will grow out of it without professional help."
- Giving advice. Advice should not be given unless chances are good that it can be applied. For example, telling a parent, "Hyperactive children need structure in their lives, such as regular mealtimes and bedtimes," would probably not be helpful to a family that lives in constant chaos.

Special Considerations for Working with Children

The health professional's approach to childhood problems differs in several important ways from the approach to adults. The first consideration is the need to work with both the parents and the child, at least until the child reaches late adolescence. The health professional usually has the advantage of a long-term relationship with the parents and familiarity with the child from an early age onward. Through periodic well-child care, the health professional develops a knowledge of the child's family and medical history and an ability to relate to parents and child alike. This background facilitates the health professional's ability to respond when social, emotional, behavioral, or learning problems emerge in the child.

The second special issue relevant to children is the necessity to view them within a developmental context. This requires a basic knowledge of the tasks of each stage of development (see Table 13.2). Further, it is essential to recognize that wide variation occurs among children within the normal range, (for example, some children may be bladder-trained at 18 months, while others aren't until after the age of three). The need to view a child within the context of his own rate of development highlights the importance of systematically recording his or her developmental milestones (for example, sitting, walking, talking, toilet training).

Awareness of differences in development among children can lead to several responses. One is that a problem is just "developmental," meaning that one should ignore the problem and give the child a chance to outgrow it. Another approach is that deviation from the norm requires immediate attention. With experience the health professional learns to observe the child for some time before getting concerned and learns when to take action.

A third special consideration is tied into the child's fluid (constantly changing) nature, which is highly responsive to environmental characteristics and events. The young child has quite limited ability to control what happens to him or her and is naturally influenced by those with the immediate responsibility for his or her welfare. Parents or guardians are in the most critical position to affect healthy growth and development in the young child. In the process of assessing problems manifested by the child, the health professional needs knowledge of the parenting provided. Many behavioral problems emanate from discipline that is either too harsh or too lenient, or from parental failure to provide the affection and love needed by children. Most often parents raise their own children the same way that they have been brought up and they have not learned that other ways might be more effective. In other instances, parents are coping with overwhelming personal problems themselves and have neither time nor emotional energy available for the child. Thus, gaining a picture from parents of their expectations of their children's behavior, as well as their re-

Table 13.2. Major Developmental Tasks of Childhood and Adolescence

Stage	Major Developmental Tasks
Infancy (birth to 3 years of age)	• Develops basic trust and sense of attachment through needs being met by parents in a predictable manner • Acquires motor skills—holds head up around 3 months, sits around 6 months, and walks in 12–18 months • Acquires speech—first word around 11–12 months with rapid vocabulary development around age 2 • Learns to manipulate objects and to play alone • Recognizes that objects are permanent even if not in sight • Begins to learn to separate from familiar persons without difficulty (strong difficulty with separating around 10–11 months and 18 months is usual) • With the ability to be mobile, becomes more independent and curious, wanting to explore everything • Expresses self often in the negative ("No" is often said by the two-year-old)—an important period for learning limits set by parents to manage aggression • Achieves bladder and bowel control (between 2 and 3 years)

Preschool (3 years to 5 years of age)	• Identification with parental models occurs, particularly with the same sex parent
	• Some understanding of right and wrong emerges
	• Acquires additional motor skills:
	    3 years old: can build a 10-cube tower; better defined drawings; jumps up and down
	    4 years old: good running, standing broad jump, and skipping; can draw a circle and a cross
	    5 years old: mature sense of balance; skips and jumps more smoothly; can copy a square and triangle
	• Learns about 50 new words a month; length of sentences increases
	• Language development includes problem-solving ability and understanding of concepts such as conservation (e.g., pouring water from tall thin container to a short wide one does not change the quantity)

continued

Table 13.2. Continued

Stage	Major Developmental Tasks
School-age (6 years through 11 years of age)	• This period has been called latency, meaning that it was considered a time of sexual inactivity, a notion that is generally not accepted today • Other authority figures than parents assume a role as the child enters school and becomes involved in social activities outside of the family • The peer group becomes important, particularly having same-sex friends • Learning, experimenting, and making things (paper dolls, kites, drawings) becomes important • Cognitive functioning increases, involving richer understanding of symbols, concepts, and rules necessary to learn to read and to handle arithmetic and other problem-solving tasks
Adolescence (12–20 years of age)	• The physical growth of adolescence, which is usually uneven, often brings with it clumsiness and hormonal changes that influence appearance, feelings, and thinking • The physical and psychological signs of adulthood begin the transition toward separation from the family and independence; in the process, conflict and turmoil are often experienced as the young person develops his or her individual identity • Major tasks during this period include completing one's education, selecting the type of work one will do, and developing a capacity to love and relate to a potential mate • An examination of values and moral standards usually occurs during this period with respect to issues such as relationships, religion, achievement and use of substances like drugs and alcohol • Changes in cognitive functioning include increased capacity for abstract thinking.

sponse to different types of behavior (successful as well as disappointing) can provide a sense of the parenting provided. While it is extremely important to avoid blaming parents for the child's problems (the child's problems are also affected by genetic, biological, and other environmental influences), it is necessary to know what kinds of parental input have influenced the child. Also, while the techniques used by parents may have been entirely successful with one sibling, another child might respond better to a different approach. Since the basics of parenting are beyond the scope of this book, the reader is referred to books by Brazelton, Wright, and Lesowitz in the resource list at the end of this chapter. Lesowitz offers some basic rules for raising children:

1. There are battles you can win and then there are those you can't win; never fight a battle you can't win.
2. Always follow through and be consistent; don't make a threat you can't keep.
3. Don't get involved with kids' behavior unless necessary; reward good behavior and ignore bad.
4. Don't put up roadblocks to kids' feelings, especially anger.
5. Don't make a kid feel like a failure; condemn the act, not the kid.
6. Set outer limits, giving kids as much freedom as possible.
7. Try to figure out what the behavior is doing for the kid.
8. Teach kids in two ways, by telling them and by showing them through example.

A fourth special consideration relevant to childhood disorders is that knowledge about these disorders is not as advanced as for adult disorders. More limited attention to child mental health services and research have contributed to this situation. The lack of a precise answer to questions about the cause or recommended treatment for a particular condition contributes to a sense of frustration on the part of the health professional, parents and children alike.

ASSESSMENT TECHNIQUES

The assessment of psychological problems and psychiatric disorders requires a knowledge of relationship-building and interviewing techniques and more technical knowledge about child development and the characteristics of specific disorders and problems that are encountered in practice. The basic strategy recommended is periodic assessment through developmental screening of all children, followed by a diagnostic conference between the health professional, parents, the child, and other key professionals, such as the child's teacher when a problem has been identified. For information about further evaluation of specific disorders, the health professional is referred to the appropriate chapter in this section and to earlier chapters for disorders common to children and adults.

Developmental Screening

In well-child visits, periodic developmental screening by the health professional is recommended to assess the child's functioning in the following areas:

1. Gross motor (e.g., sitting, crawling, walking, climbing)
2. Fine motor (e.g., building with blocks, picking up small items)
3. Speech and language (e.g., spoken words, understanding of sounds)
4. Social behavior (e.g., imitative behavior, play)

Instruments such as the Denver Developmental Screening Test* can be efficiently administered in about 15 minutes for infants and preschoolers, and has good reliability until age four. Age-normative data are provided, along with some guidelines indicating when deviation represents cause for further evaluation.

The absence of widely accepted screening measures for the school-age child or adolescent requires that the health professional rely on his or her judgment about age-appropriateness of the behavior exhibited by a particular child. Major developmental tasks, as outlined in Table 13.2, may vary across cultures, socioeconomic classes, and among individual children within specific cultural or socioeconomic groups.

Developmental screening, whether conducted with a formal instrument, such as the Denver Developmental Screening Test, or through interview, usually benefits from two sources of data. The parent will be asked to report on behavior that is not easily observable in the office, and the child can be directly evaluated in the office on other tasks. As much direct assessment of the child as possible is recommended, since parents may present a biased report of the child's functioning.

The health professional will need some simple equipment in the office, if only for the purpose of establishing rapport with a child. Examples of items that should be on hand include paper and pencil (or crayons), a ball, a simple puzzle, dolls, and several children's books with pictures. The child can be helped to feel at ease through being offered play activities, and such materials can be easily used to assess different types of functioning. For example, the paper and crayons can be used to ask a child to draw a picture of himself and/or his family, which provides some measure of his ability level and his self-concept. The drawings in Figure 1 represent average ability for each age group. The drawing with the tiny child in the corner may indicate a negative self-concept or fearfulness. To use such drawings for assessing psychological perceptions and intellectual functioning, the reader is referred to D. B. Harris' book in the resource references at the end of this chapter.

An outline for the assessment process follows:

---

*Developed by William K. Frankenburg, M. D., and Josiah B. Dodds, Ph.D., of the University of Colorado Medical Center; it is distributed in the United States by the Mead Johnson Laboratory.

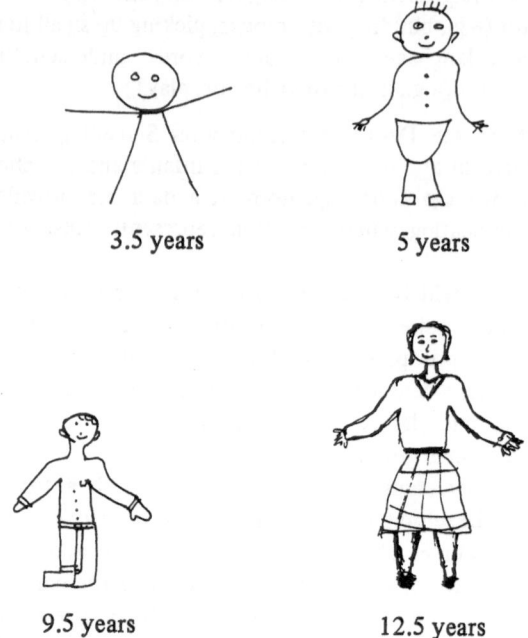

3.5 years   5 years

9.5 years   12.5 years

Figure 13.1.   Examples of average-ability child drawings of self.

1. Take a complete medical history.
2. Take a developmental history, obtaining the child's age for critical milestones.
3. Get information on the family background and relationships between family members.
4. Get a report of school functioning.
5. Obtain a description of the behavioral or emotional problem as seen by the parents, including information on the duration of the problem and the circumstances under which it occurs.
6. Ask parents what type of assistance they expect from the health professional.

CLINICAL MANAGEMENT

Although the steps for managing specific problems and disorders are described in each section on specific problems or disorders, there are some general principles that apply to most problems presented to the health professional.

Prevention

1. Give anticipatory guidance to parents on problems common to all children (e.g., procedures and age for toilet-training)
2. Educate parents about normal growth and development
3. Give parents a chance to express their own concerns about new experiences (e.g., fears about the first baby or concerns about sending the child off to school for the first time).

Supportive Counseling

1. Include parents, unless an adolescent (patient) has actually declared independence and is out of the household.
2. Allow parents and the child to present their concerns without your interrupting or making judgments.
3. Focus on strengthening parents' functioning regarding the child.
4. Work with parents to modify negative attitudes toward the child.
5. Help parents develop specific goals for themselves and the child, along with a plan to pursue them.
6. Help parents understand that the problem did not develop overnight and that change may be slow, but encourage them to look for small signs of change.

LIFE CRISES AND OTHER PSYCHOLOGICAL PROBLEMS

There are a number of problems experienced by children in the course of living that may be temporarily stressful or that may develop into more serious or prolonged disorders, such as those described in the subsequent chapters. The health professional is in a good position to take preventive action to alleviate distress at an early stage and thereby prevent more serious consequences at a later stage. Although some of these problems have a course that may not be altered (e.g., a chronic medical illness), attention to psychological aspects can facilitate better adjustment or adaptation to such afflictions. For the following problems, the health professional can assume at least an educational and supportive counseling role.

Birth of a Sibling

The birth of a sibling is a normal event, but it may create a sense of discomfort in the child. This event can be usually handled through preparatory steps such as talking with the child about the expected arrival of a new brother or sister. Because of changed cultural attitudes about birth as a family event, young children are now often able to see the new sibling soon after birth, instead of having to spend several days worrying about the mother and the new baby. When the baby comes home, the older sibling is likely to need special attention to reassure him that his special place in the family has not been lost. Indications that the child may have such feelings are often observed in regressive behavior, such as wanting a bottle for milk or bed-wetting in the child who has stayed dry through the night for some time.

Hospitalization

Hospitalization of a child may evoke fears about separation from parents, fears about his or her illness (sometimes thought of as punishment for bad behavior), or fearfulness about medical or surgical procedures. Again, proper preparation is the key to reducing such concerns. The health professional, in addition to talking with the child and parents about what to expect, can also help the preschool or school-age child to play out the coming experience with doctor and nurse dolls. The parents can be encouraged to help the child to talk at home and to play with a doctor or nurse kit. A preliminary visit to the hospital to see the ward and play room is also recommended. In addition, letting the child know when parents will visit him or her at the hospital is helpful. Some hospitals offer parents the opportunity to live in the same room with the child. While this practice may not be possible (for example, the parent may need to care for other children at home), having a parent live in the hospital can be reassuring when the child is in considerable pain or going through a variety of procedures that are unfamiliar. The presence of a parent as the child comes out of recovery from surgery is important, and should be arranged if at all possible.

Parent-Child Conflict

Conflict is normal in the process of the child's achieving independence and the parents' enforcing certain limits; however, constant struggle between parents and children reduces the chances of gratification for either group. The health professional can help assess whether the conflict is generated by normal development (e.g., the "no" stage of the two-year-old or independence-seeking behavior of an adolescent); by unmet needs of the parent (who may be overly controlling); or by a behavioral disorder in the child. The preceding situations are dealt with differently. If the problem is developmental, simply providing reassurance that the stage will pass if not too much of an issue is made is usually sufficient. Parents can be taught to direct the child from unwanted behavior or, in the case of an adolescent, they can give credit where independence has truly been achieved. The overly harsh, strict, or controlling parent, who may see the child as a miniature adult, may need help with reducing expectations appropriate to the child's developmental stage. In many cases, the conflict starts around an issue like toilet-training, and, if recognized by the health professional at an early point, much subsequent grief can be spared. Parents who provide little control for children or fail to set limits at all end up in conflict with children who are acting out to elicit attention. Such parents may need help in examining their priorities and identifying ways to obtain sufficient time and emotional energy to relate to the child or children. The latter recommendation is not easy for parents in situations in which both parents have to work, in which a single parent is solely responsible for raising children, or when parents have emotional problems of their own, thus requiring extra patience and support from the health professional.

In cases where the parenting seems to be adequate and the child's conduct is problematic, it is important to find out whether the child has been through a recent traumatic event that might explain a change in his or her relationship with parents. Giving the child a chance to talk about the event, express feelings and get some understanding can lead to changed behavior.

Aggressive Behavior

Some children are in frequent conflict with parents, school authorities, or others in the neighborhood. Such children may be described as stubborn, difficult, or oppositional. The basis may lie in problems with parenting as described above, in cultural values that reward behavior such as stealing, or in a specific disorder in the child. The initial focus on parenting should address issues such as whether expectations or behavioral limits are clearly established by parents and whether the parental response to the child is consistent (e.g., do parents threaten punishment and then ignore the behavior?). In the case where the child is merely conforming to neighborhood norms (for example, if constant fighting and rough play are engaged in by all children in the area), then environmental manipulation, like sending the child to a different school or moving to a different community, may be necessary. If efforts directed toward altering the parents' behavior or the environment do not result in improved behavior in the child, the next step is to assess whether one of the childhood disorders may be the problem. For example, a child with mental retardation, hyperactivity, learning disabilities, or conduct disorders may not understand directions given or he or she may not have developed the internal controls necessary to direct his or her behavior.

Shy Behavior

The shy or withdrawn child is less likely to receive special attention, because such behavior does not bother others and is therefore not viewed as a problem. There are many quiet children whose adjustment is entirely adequate; they are not the concern of this section. However, in the case of the child who finds it painful to answer a question in class or to enter into play with other children, there is a legitimate need for investigation. Questions such as whether the child has been overpowered by older siblings or been through frightening experiences (for example, being raised in a family with a lot of loud arguing) need to be raised. (If the child seems to have real fears about separating from parents or going to school, see Chapter 17, "Anxiety Disorders of Childhood.") Most of these children will respond to individual attention and encouragement. An example of a plan for a shy child would be to observe his or her difficulties and find strengths that can be used to involve him or her with other children. Making fun of the child or pressuring him or her to become more outgoing will not succeed. If the child is extremely withdrawn and has little or no language by age five, see Chapter 19, "Mental Retardation," and Chapter 15, "Specific Developmental Disorders" (language disabilities section). In the case of extreme but rare behavior in which there is no communication with the child (possibility of childhood autism), referred to a mental health specialist is essential.

Academic Problems

Learning or school achievement problems are quite common and are difficult to assess, since they can stem from many different reasons. The parent is likely to learn from the school by way of a report card or a special note that the child is not achieving up to the standard of his classmates. This may occur as early as preschool or kindergarten, if the child does not seem to have mastered the readiness skills for reading and writing that will be taught in first grade. More commonly, such children are not identified until third or fourth grade when the material becomes more difficult to master and the child is lacking the basic skills that should have been acquired in the first and second years of school. The family may seek assistance from the health professional in determining the cause of the problem. Table 13.3 may be used by the health professional for the initial assessment and intervention in academic problems.

Separation and Divorce

Many children today come from families in which the parents are separated or have gotten a divorce, which was preceded by years of conflict or tension. Three major issues that can have an emotional or social impact on the child of such a family are:

- Feelings of responsibility for the parents' splitting up;
- Guilt feelings about loyalty and positive feelings toward one or the other parent;
- A sense of loss, missing the parent who is not at home with child.

The health professional can help parents to avoid blaming the child for any role in the dissolution of the marriage and to avoid using the child as a weapon to hurt each other. In many instances the child gets caught in the conflict between the parents and serves as a vehicle for aggression by being manipulative (e.g., the child may tell the mother about the father's young girlfriend). Although conflict within the marriage may have centered around management of the children, they are not responsible for the parents' inability to be compatible. The health professional can help each parent avoid criticizing the other parent in front of the child. Whatever the failings of either parent, the child needs to come to his or her own judgment about each parent and needs to be free to maintain previously established emotional bonds. In order to avoid a great sense of loss, the child needs to have regular contact with the parent who no longer resides in the home. This is obviously problematic if the other parent has moved out of town or cannot visit the children regularly for whatever reason. Some contact, if desired by the child, can still be kept up through correspondence or occasional visits. Prohibiting contact may result in destructive behavior on the child's part (e.g., criminal acts with the expectation of joining the missing father in prison). Just because the parent has not been an adequate marital partner or even an acceptable member of society does not negate a child's feelings towards him or her.

Loss of a Parent or Sibling

Loss through death of a parent, sibling, or friend is difficult for a child at any age. The younger the child, the greater likelihood that the child will not understand for some time what has really occurred. The younger child (preschool) may think that the parent has just gone away and will return in a few days. Involving the child in the usual family rituals around death helps him or her take in the meaning of the event, while exclusion may lead to a greater sense of mystery and fantasies that are longer-lasting. It is important for the child to observe feelings of grief and loss felt by other members of the family, thereby allowing him or her to feel sad too. At the same time it is important to provide assurance that he or she will continue to be cared for and looked after. In the weeks and months after the death, it is important to answer the child's questions about the person who has died and to provide opportunities to talk about positive memories as well as to express feelings of sadness and loss. The health professional can encourage the preceding by scheduling a visit shortly after the death, during which it is possible to discuss such matters as the advisability of the child's attending the funeral or going to the cemetery, and then can schedule another visit a few months later.

Table 13.3. Initial Assessment Plan for Academic Problems

Basis of Learning Problem	Description	Health Professional's Role
Immaturity. Seen usually before the age of 8; may have physiological basis or result from insufficient stimulation by parents in early years	Child has difficulty settling down to sedentary tasks, shows little interest in tasks, and would prefer to engage in more active play.	Assess neurophysiological development; if child is not ready for required learning tasks, consider remedial help or placement in a lower grade if child is beyond kindergarten.
Emotional conflict; recent stress such as separation of parents.	In a child who usually performs daydreaming in class, acting out by speaking out of turn, and failure to work.	Identify nature of problem and provide supportive counseling.
Personality conflict with teacher. Teacher's style of relating to child is different from parents or previous teacher	Child constantly in conflict with teacher over requirements, both academic and behavioral.	Work with child and parents on adjusting to teacher's requirements; if not successful, request a conference with the teacher and school officials to review problem and attempt to find solutions; if that is not feasible, request assignment to a different teacher.
Hyperactivity	Child fails to pay attention, constantly moves, doesn't complete assignments.	(See Chapter 14 of this book, "Hyperactivity.")

Learning disabilities	Inconsistent performance; child does well in some areas and poorly in others.	See Chapter 15 of this book, "Specific Developmental Disorders (Learning Disabilities)."
Mental retardation	Child has difficulty in all academic subjects.	See Chapter 19 of this book, "Mental Retardation."
Medical condition (e.g., poor sight, poor hearing, anemia)	Child with prior history of adequate achievement falls behind without apparent reason.	Conduct a complete physical examination.
Other emotional disorder	Child lacks energy or interest, gets tearful easily. Child is afraid to answer in class but performs well on written tasks.	See Chapter 5, "Syndrome of Depression," or Chapter 17, "Anxiety Disorders of Childhood."
Environmental problems (e.g., malnutrition associated with poverty or junk food and soft beverages diet, or minimal sleep due to poor housing)	Achievement generally low; no particular behavioral pattern.	Home visit recommended; help from social services very useful; also work with school personnel to obtain remedial educational assistance.
Home environment— minimal or inadequate parental attention to child's schoolwork	Child has ability but refuses to do school work; does not bring in homework; does not appear interested in school.	Provide specific instruction for parents to encourage child's schoolwork and to ensure that homework is completed before play time.

Child Neglect and Abuse

This is a more common problem than most people suspect and one that is likely to come to the attention of the health professional in the hospital emergency room or in outpatient practice. The child is brought in with explanations of an accidental fall when he has been dropped or thrown. Other children are noticed during routine pediatric care because of unexplainable bruises or burns on their bodies. It is difficult to get parents to admit responsibility for injuries because of the shame associated with neglecting or harming one's own child, as well as fear of legal consequences (e.g., that the child will be taken away and placed in foster care). Also, the health professional's anger towards the parents may interfere with communicating effectively with them. Making clear to the parents that your role is to help both the child and parents is the first step.

Next, it is important to get a complete history of the abusive behavior to assess further risk to the child. Under what conditions has the abuse occurred? Was it following alcohol use, conflict between husband and wife, certain provocative or stubborn behavior on the part of the child, a general sense of being overwhelmed with the responsibilities of parenting, or was it associated with other economic or emotional problems? Was the abusing parent abused as a child? (Abusing parents usually have a history of being abused themselves.) Keep in mind that hyperactive or otherwise handicapped children are at higher risk of being abused than are average children.

After assessment of abusing behavior, the next task is to assess whether the parent has a way to stop his or her behavior when he or she feels that he or she may hurt the child. Once the parents start to open up, in addition to feelings of anger and guilt, they express fears about their ability to hurt their child, feelings not terribly apparent when parents deny any involvement in the injuries. The health professional should try to present a plan for preventing abusive behavior when parents feel out of control and try to get them to agree to contact a helping organization when in danger. Many cities have hotlines where parents can call in and get immediate help over the telephone. If the preceding is achieved, then sending the child home with a plan for further follow-up may be appropriate.

The preceding professional judgment is an extremely difficult one to make and the health professional may want to call on a mental health or social services specialist to help assess this. If, on the other hand, the child has been seriously injured and requires hospitalization, time to observe child-parent interactions and to call in other specialists will create the opportunity to come up with a more thoroughly considered long-term plan. If the child is moderately injured and parents do not think they can control their behavior (e.g., "the next time the child pours his milk on the floor, I will kill him"), there is no choice but to arrange for an immediate emergency placement. In some instances, this might involve a temporary stay with a relative who lives nearby. If parents are embarrassed about family members' learning about the problem, placement in an emergency shelter for abused children, usually a group home under the auspices of the local Welfare Department, or in a foster home should be considered. Local legislation spells out the legal requirements for reporting child abuse, and health professionals must be knowledgeable about any legal provisions. Child abuse can be life-threatening.

Obesity

Although obesity may be considered a medical rather than psychological problem, its roots are very often psychological in nature. The rationale for overfeeding or poor nutrition may be cultural ("a fat baby is a loved baby"); poor dietary habits based on misunderstanding of dietary needs or inability to afford a balanced diet; or substitution of food for love. For the overweight child, eating is a major source of pleasure. In many cultures, such children lose out on positive social experiences. The "fat" child may be teased, excluded from sports and, as a teenager, may experience peer group rejection and limited relationships with the opposite sex. The health professional's role is to intervene early in the dietary habits of the mother during pregnancy and then to carefully monitor the child's weight in relation to his growth. Fat cells develop very early in life and retain the obesity traits, which are extremely difficult to eliminate in later life. Therefore, where obesity seems to be a problem in the family, intensive nutritional education of parents is strongly recommended. When an overweight child is not identified until school age, it is important to work with the parents and child together to develop a sensible dietary program, which will have a long-term effect. This involves balancing the diet with the basic food types and slowly cutting back on foods like carbohydrates that will contribute to further weight gain. Extreme diets (e.g., cottage cheese and grapefruit) are not recommended as they do not change overall eating habits on a long-term basis and can also lead to other medical conditions due to nutritional imbalances. Getting the overweight child or adolescent involved in an exercise program—preferably swimming, walking, or a sport that he or she can enjoy—is also strongly recommended. If the health professional doesn't start to get some results after several months, referral to a nutritionist for individual or group counseling may be quite important. Since parents are likely to accept the expertise of the health professional regarding obesity, early intervention has a good chance of achieving weight loss and preventing later psychological problems and medical conditions.

Chronic and Fatal Medical Conditions

Chronic medical conditions present psychological problems because of associated behavioral handicaps or impairments (e.g., blindness) or because of the life-threatening nature of certain conditions (e.g., cancer). With the discovery of a condition such as a birth defect or a serious illness, the health professional needs to be carefully tuned in to the parents' feelings. Despite a clear description of the diagnosis, the expected course of the condition, and treatment, parents are likely to recall a very limited amount of what they were told in a first session. Several sessions will be needed to review and repeat information as parents tend to go through a grieving process. The initial reaction may be one of numbness and shock, followed by a sense of disbelief and a search for other explanations. During this stage it is important that the health professional not get angry when the parents take the child to other doctors or hospitals to disconfirm the diagnosis or to seek a magical cure. Next comes anger, which may be directed at the health professional for failure to make an earlier diagnosis or towards the parents themselves. Despair, or a sense that the future will be even worse, is finally followed by a sense of acceptance, at which time it becomes possible to develop a plan to make the best of the situation for parents and child alike. These stages don't follow a firm pattern, and some of them may be repeated when there is a setback in the child or difficulty in paying the necessary medical bills.

As time goes on, further problems, such as the effect on other siblings or the isolation of the family, become apparent and the family can benefit from the guidance of the health professional. What and how much to tell the child varies with his or her age and maturity. In addition, the ill child needs opportunities to express his feelings and fears as well as a chance to develop as normally as possible, both socially and educationally. The emotional needs of the child, the parents and other family members will require regularly scheduled sessions with the health professional. Since the specific needs vary with the type of condition that the child has, the reader is referred to a very helpful book by Richard Lansdown (1980), *More than Sympathy*, which recommends approaches to eight handicapping conditions and seven life-threatening conditions.

Problems of Adolescence

Adolescence has been portrayed as a period of conflict and struggle as the young person moves toward independence from the family and begins to make major life decisions. In societies that ritualize this stage through well-defined tasks, this stage of development seems to be less traumatic. In Western societies, where there is considerable variation in the age of marriage, completing one's education, and beginning employment, the adolescent may spend many years in a role that is neither fully child nor adult. Experimentation with taking on adult behaviors is integral to becoming a full-fledged adult. However, in some areas the adolescent may not be prepared to accept the responsibility that comes with sexual experience or consumption of alcohol or drugs. While experimentation is normal, such behaviors may be influenced by factors such as peer pressure, by unhappiness, or by conflicts with parents that result in rebellious behavior.

The adolescent's relationship with a health professional can offer an opportunity to explore feelings and experiences and to obtain information, thus potentially preventing more serious problems. For the young person in trouble it is very important to have access to an accepting professional. If the adolescent feels that the health professional will be judgmental, he or she is not likely to open up about drug use, venereal disease, alcohol abuse, or other serious concerns.

Pregnancy prior to marriage is frequently seen by health providers. Below we provide some suggestions for responding to a possible pregnancy:

1. During regular health maintenance visits, give teens a chance to talk about sexual experiences and relationships; provide education as needed.
2. When a young female says that she might be pregnant,
   - Review her recent sexual behavior to assess the feasibility of pregnancy;
   - Review her knowledge about birth control and any birth control practices used;
   - Ask how the patient feels about the possibility of a pregnancy. Some will be very anxious and unhappy, while others will feel good about having a child, even though the HP may have difficulty understanding that a fourteen-year-old wants to become a parent;
   - Confirm whether or not the patient is pregnant;
   - If she is pregnant, ask the patient what her intentions are. Does she expect to follow through with the pregnancy and if so, does she plan to keep the child?
   - Find out who else knows about the pregnancy—the patient's parents, the father of the child, friends—and what their feelings are. It is essential to ensure that some people in the patient's life are available to provide emotional support, as an unplanned pregnancy may lead to feelings of anxiety and/or depression;
   - Depending on the availability of supportive people in the patient's life and the age of the patient, consider a session with the patient and one of her parents to discuss plans for the pregnancy. Many young women who protest about presenting their situation are quite relieved when this has been accomplished, particularly when this can occur with the health professional present;
   - Schedule follow-up appointments to discuss the many decisions that will have to be made and to keep in touch with the patient's feelings. This supportive counseling can be incorporated into prenatal visits;
   - If abortion occurs, there are often psychological consequences usually manifested as a feeling of loss and other depressive symptoms which may necessitate follow-up counseling.

- In the event that such a child is given for adoption, supportive counseling may be an important function of the health professional.
- Start counseling to prevent a second pregnancy long before the patient is able to conceive again—a second unplanned pregnancy is not unusual;
- Throughout the pregnancy it is important to help the teen-ager explore other goals, such as education or work. In many areas, the pregnant teen-ager can continue to attend school or can go to a special educational program for pregnant teen-agers;
- Special follow-up sessions after pregnancy (whether it was terminated, the baby was given up for adoption, or it was kept) are needed to assess psychological adjustment.

REFERENCES

Brazelton TB. *Infants and Mothers: Differences in Development.* New York: Delacorte Press, 1969.

Brazelton TB. *Toddlers and Parents: A Declaration of Independence.* New York: Delacorte Press, 1974.

Fraiberg SH. *The Magic Years: Understanding and Handling the Problems of Early Childhood.* New York: Scribner, 1959.

Harris DB. *Children's Drawings as Measures of Mental Maturity.* New York: Harcourt, Brace, World, 1963.

Justice B, Justice R. *The Abusing Family.* New York: Human Sciences Press, 1976.

Lansdown R. *More Than Sympathy.* London: Tavistock Publications, 1980.

Lesowitz RI. *Rules for Raising Kids.* Springfield, Ill.: Charles C Thomas Co., 1974.

Shafil M, Shafil SL. *Pathways of Human Development.* New York: Thieme-Stratton, Inc., 1982.

Simmons JE. *Psychiatric Examination of Children,* 3rd Ed. Philadelphia: Lea and Febiger, 1981.

Wright L. *Parent Power: a Guide to Responsible Child Rearing.* New York: Morrow, 1980.

CHAPTER 14

Hyperactivity
(Attention Deficit Disorder)

The child who suffers from hyperactivity has been described as someone "who consistently exhibits a high level of activity in situations in which it is clearly inappropriate, is unable to inhibit his activity on command, often appears capable of only one speed of response and is often characterized by other physiological, learning and behavioral symptoms and problems" (Werry and Sprague, 1970). The cause is still largely debated, although genetic, neurological, developmental, and environmental explanations have been offered. Incidence is reported from 4% to 20% among schoolage children. The disorder is much more common among boys than girls (in a ratio of 4 to 1), and the chances of identifying the problem are largely a function of the disruption that the child creates for parents and teachers.

CLINICAL PICTURE

The activity of the hyperactive child is not only excessive, but frequently purposeless or lacking in goal orientation. Hyperactivity, also known by other terms such as minimal brain dysfunction and hyperkinesis, has been identified most recently as one component of the attention deficit disorder. From this point on in our discussion, each time a reference is made to hyperactivity, both activity and attention problems are understood to be included, as well as impulsivity. Attention problems refer to an inability to focus on or stay with a specific activity. The child with an attention deficit disorder, in addition to hyperactivity, displays signs of developmentally inappropriate attention and impulsivity for his or her mental and chronological age. Attention problems are manifested in behaviors such as difficulty concentrating on schoolwork or completing a game. Impulsive behavior is usually described as acting before thinking.

Hyperactivity is sometimes observable at birth; the child is more fidgety and active than others. However, some children are very quiet as infants and their hyperactivity does not become evident until the child walks and seems to get into everything. In others, hyperactivity is not observable until entry into school, where children are expected to be able to sit quietly in most cultures. For many children hyperactivity will remit spontaneously around age 8, when neurological development is sufficiently advanced to allow control of motor and cognitive behavior. Recent studies have indicated that for a number of hyperactive children, the disorder continues into adolescence or even adulthood. The degree of later adjustment seems to be related to the intellectual ability of the child. The brighter the child, the more likely that he or she will learn to handle his or her activity level, problems with paying attention, or impulsive behavior.

It is important to note that behavioral symptoms of hyperactivity are not manifested consistently in all situations. They occur on some occasions but are absent on others. Symptoms diminish in one-to-one relationships and in highly structured situations, but increase in group and less structured environments. In addition, hyperactive children frequently evidence an uneven developmental profile. For example, they excel in gross motor areas, while showing delay in fine motor skills; or the opposite may be true. Hyperactive children are often physically and socially attractive, and may have a special ability to develop affectionate relationships, despite their problematic behaviors.

DIAGNOSIS

Hyperactivity or attention deficit disorder can be assessed by the Questionnaire for Hyperactivity given below.

QUESTIONNAIRE FOR HYPERACTIVITY*

(To be given to parents)

Contact with the child's teacher by either the health professional or the parents may be necessary to answer certain questions about the child's behavior in school. The questions are to be answered YES or NO; the scores of each subgroup (i.e., Inattention + 3, Impulsivity + 3, and Hyperactivity + 2) provide

---

*Adapted from DSM-III.

criteria for diagnosis. If the Hyperactivity score is less than 2, then the diagnosis
is Attention Deficit Disorder without hyperactivity.

	YES	NO

A. *Inattention:*

1. Does the child tend to leave things unfinished (e.g.,
   homework, school assignments)?

2. Do you usually have to make a request 3 or 4 times
   before you get a response?

3. Do you have to tell the child that he or she does not
   pay close enough attention to the job or tasks that he
   or she is asked to do?

4. Does the child have trouble keeping his or her mind
   on an assignment at school?

5. Does the child have trouble sticking with play activities (e.g., watching T.V., playing games)?

B. *Impulsivity:*

1. Does the child tend to get into trouble or hurt because he or she rushed into something without thinking
   what might happen?

2. Does the child tend to hurry from one activity to
   another, before finishing the first one?

3. Does the child have difficulties organizing work at
   home or at school?

4. Do you have to tell the child repeatedly what to do?

5. Does the child get into trouble at school because of
   speaking out when he or she is supposed to be quiet;

6. When playing or lining up, does the child *often* try
   to get ahead of others for his or her turn?

C. *Hyperactivity :*

1. Is the child always on the move or does he or she act
   as if driven by a motor?

2. Does the child have difficulty sitting still without
   fidgeting?

3. Does the child have difficulty staying seated at
   school?

4. Does he or she move excessively during sleep?

Differential Diagnosis

Anxiety

An attention deficit disorder with hyperactivity can be a secondary symptom of anxiety. The presence of some of the signs and symptoms of anxiety such as fearful expectations, fearful attitude, overconcern about daily events (e.g., parents going out at night), repetitive nightmares, and difficulty in tolerating stress might suggest the presence of an overanxious disorder. (See Chapter 17, "Anxiety Disorders of Childhood.")

Depression

Depression can also be associated with hyperactivity and attention deficit disorder. The specific elements of the disorder should be carefully investigated. (See Chapter 5, "The Syndrome of Depression"). One problem with depressive symptoms, pointed out by some researchers, is that they can be a result of the hyperactivity.

Conduct disorders

Conduct disorders can also be confused with attention deficit disorder, but the behavioral considerations are clearly secondary while the obvious transgression of social norms, lack of consideration for others, the absence of guilt feelings, and the lack of responsibility, constitute the primary considerations in conduct disorders. (See Chapter 16, "Conduct Disorders.")

A neurological disorder

A neurological disorder such as epilepsy, the sequelae of encephalitis, congenital cerebral malformation, and other obvious organic factors affecting the central nervous system can be associated with hyperactivity and should be ruled out before the primary diagnosis of hyperactivity or attention deficit disorder is made.

CLINICAL MANAGEMENT

Have parents provide a complete diagnostic history of the child (see Chapter 3, "The History"). At the same time, help them to discuss any guilt feelings, anger, and despair about the child's problem. Be supportive and understanding, focus on the positive aspects of the relationship with the child (i.e., try to identify how specific responses to the child's behavior have been effective). Through this process, parents will be stimulated to work further with the child. The goal

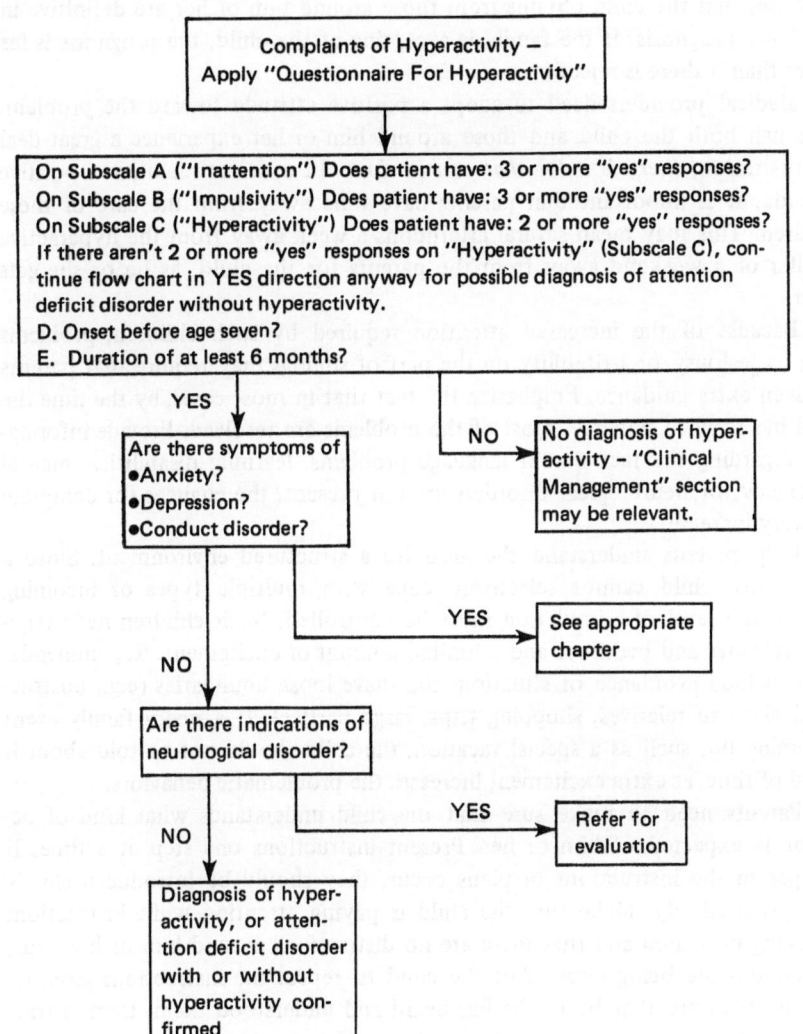

Figure 14.1. Attention deficit disorder with hyperactivity, diagnostic flow chart.

is to provide behavioral control, while expecting gradual internalization of learning on the part of the child.

It is essential to focus the treatment procedures not exclusively on the child, but on interrelationships between child, parents, and teachers, since the responses that the child obtains from those around him or her are definitive in his or her prognosis. If the family is accepting of the child, the prognosis is far better than if there is rejection.

Medical providers need to adopt a positive attitude toward the problem. Although both the child and those around him or her experience a great deal of frustration, *there is a lot that can be done.* In order to maintain a positive attitude, it is important that parents have time away from the care of these children. This may mean several afternoons a week away from the hyperactive toddler or a weekend away from the parents for the child, as he or she gets older.

Because of the increased attention required by such children, problems such as jealousy or irritability on the part of siblings may require that parents be given extra guidance. Emphasize the fact that in most cases, by the time the child has reached puberty, most of the problems are resolved. Provide information regarding the fact that if language problems, learning disabilities, mental deficiency, or neurological disorders are not present, the chances for complete recovery increase.

Help parents understand the need for a structured environment. Since a hyperactive child cannot selectively cope with multiple types of incoming stimuli, the level of stimulation must be controlled. Such children need regular mealtimes and bedtimes and a limited amount of excitement. Recommendations include avoidance of situations that have loose boundaries (e.g., unstructured visits to relatives, shopping trips, large parties). If a major family event is coming up, such as a special vacation, the child should not be told about it ahead of time, as extra excitement increases the problematic behaviors.

Parents need to make sure that the child understands what kind of behavior is expected of him or her. Present instructions one step at a time. If changes in the instructions or plans occur, they should be introduced slowly and systematically. Make sure the child is paying attention while instructions are being presented and that there are no distractions around him or her while instructions are being given. Ask the child to repeat the instructions given by parents to assure that he or she has heard and understood them. Demonstrate repeatedly the advantages of waiting or slowing down.

One source of support for parents may be a local group of parents who meet to discuss management strategies. Parents provide emotional support to each other as well as offer helpful tips for handling the child's troublesome behaviors.

Consultation by the health professional with the school is also important. Teachers need to understand that the child's behavior is not purposeful, and that providing structure similar to that at home is important (e.g., it may be necessary to have the child sit in the front area of the classroom near the teacher). The preceding steps should be completed over a two- to four-week period. If unsuccessful, consider the use of psychotropic medication.

Drug Treatment

Drug treatment with central nervous system stimulants for attention deficit disorders with hyperactivity is a frequent, although debated, therapeutic approach. Once the disorder is diagnosed and the preceding steps have been attempted, the child can be started on a medication trial. The goal of treatment is to find out the right dosage that helps the child control unwanted symptoms. The purpose of the medication should be explained to the child and relatives. The aim of treatment is not to oversedate the child, but to help him or her control unproductive behavior such that he is able to learn in school and to exert some control over his behavior at home. There are three drugs discussed that may be used in children over 6 years of age: dextroamphetamine sulfate, racemic amphetamine, and methylphenidate hydrochloride.

Dextroamphetamine sulfate

Presentation: 5 mg/tablets. Initial trial: 2.5 mg in the morning for one week to test side effects and tolerance; afterwards increase by 5 mg weekly until optimum results are achieved—to no more than 40 mg/day. Use before breakfast and before lunch and be aware of potential side effects: insomnia, headache, dryness of the mouth, loss of appetite, and tachycardia. Irritability, tenseness, or obvious sedation may be observed in the course of the treatment if the dosage is excessive. A decrease in medication or discontinuation of treatment is then suggested. Sustained-release capsules are available in 5 mg, 10 mg and 15 mg, which eliminates a second daily administration of medication.

Racemic amphetamine

May be used in identical presentations, dosages, and uses as for dextroamphetamine; side effects are also similar. In some cases, individual reactions to one drug are not consistent with another drug; therefore, a trial of different medications is worthwhile when side effects are a problem.

Methylphenidate hydrochloride

Presentation: 5 mg, 10 mg, and 20 mg/tablets; a similar procedure to the one used for the amphetamines may be used with methylphenidate hydrochloride, except that weekly increase can be up to 10 mg. Daily dosages above 60 mg are not recommended. This is also available in a sustained release capsule.

For all these drugs it can be said that a one- to two-month trial period would be desirable before discontinuation, which would occur if no beneficial effects are seen and the maximum dosages have been kept up for at least one month. Treatment-resistant cases (those without results after a month of treatment compliance) should be referred to the mental health specialist. If the drug proves to be helpful, it should be used for 6 months to a year with occasional drug-free periods after the first 6 months of continuous treatment. If during the

Table 14.1. Attention Deficit Disorder with Hyperactivity, Management

Spend 4 weeks in the following 8 steps

1. Obtain clinical history from parents and school. Explore guilt, anger, frustration in parents.
2. Focus treatment on interrelationships among child-parents-teacher, not exclusively on the child.
3. Encourage positive attitude toward change to foster good prognosis.
4. Encourage parents to spend time away from child.
5. Emphasize the importance of a structured environment.
6. Communicate expectations of child to him or her slowly and clearly; avoid giving multiple instructions at one time.
7. Encourage parental involvement in a parent support group.
8. Consult with school personnel.

If there is no improvement after 4 weeks and the child is over 6 years of age,* consider:

9. Drug treatment:
   • Explain the rationale of drug treatment to child and relatives.
   • De-emphasize its importance by emphasizing 1 through 8.
   • Use before breakfast and before lunch dosages or single dose in sustained-release capsule.
   • Start with:
     Dextroamphetamine sulfate or Racemic amphetamine
     5 mg/tablets; initial 2.5 mg/day/one week, then
     5 mg/day/with 5-mg increments weekly—maximum dosage related to child's weight—careful attention to side effects (use 2 daily doses)
     Alternative drug: Methylphenidate hydrochloride: similar dosages
   • Careful attention to side effects (i.e., irritability, tenseness; sedation)
   • Keep administering drugs from 6 months to 1 year
   • If during drug-free periods there is no recurrence of hyperactive or ADD behavior, discontinue drug treatment.
10. Refer to a mental health specialist if there is no improvement after a trial period of one to two months.
11. Reassess the child's progress periodically and provide continued support and guidance to parents.

*In extreme cases, consider drug treatment at an earlier age, but *not before three years of age.*

drug-free periods there is a recurrence of symptomatology, the treatment should be initiated again in the same form as stated. For all three above-mentioned drugs, regular monitoring of the child's height and weight gain is important.

Behavior modification techniques usually constitute the psychologist's or educational specialist's field of expertise. Some of them include: techniques in a classroom routine that allow maximum physical movement; a token economy system (tokens are given for targeted behaviors, which can later be exchanged for rewards such as food, toys, or special privileges); and a combination of reinforcers and a highly structured, directive teaching program to reduce rough physical behavior. These and related procedures are normally handled by specialists to whom hyperactive children will have to be referred. Educational personnel typically assess the child's capabilities, sensory or otherwise, and work to build a program around the child's stronger areas. See Chapter 15, "Specific Developmental Disorders, (Learning Disabilities)." Parents can also use information about the child's strengths in working with their child.

If the management approaches described above do not result in observable improvement, then referral to a mental health or special education specialist is advisable. The first step is likely to consist of further evaluation of the child to assess strengths and to look for related problems such as learning disabilities (see Chapter 15). Mental health specialists or special education specialists may recommend behavior modification approaches, which can be implemented both at home and at school. Such approaches might include a reinforcement program to recognize desired behavior (e.g., a small reward for longer periods of attending to one task).

Whether the child is referred to a specialist or followed exclusively by the health professional, periodic reassessment by the health professional is important. As such children grow larger and stronger, they are likely to engage in activities that are more worrisome to parents (e.g., the impulsive four-year old starts the family automobile). Parents need support and guidance on a regular basis. While they can use practical advice about how to respond to specific behavioral problems, they also need recognition for the difficult task of parenting hyperactive children on a 24-hour basis. Exceptional patience is required to avoid getting angry at a child who never finishes anything, doesn't go to sleep until late at night and gets up early as well, and who can manage to put a house in disarray in five minutes!

REFERENCE

Laufer MW, Shett Taranath S. Attention Deficit Disorders. In: *Comprehensive Textbook of Psychiatry*, Kaplan HI, Freedman AM, Sadock BJ (Eds.). Baltimore: Williams and Wilkins Co., 1980.

Wender P. *Minimal Brain Dysfunction in Children*. New York: Wiley-Interscience, 1971.

Werry JS, Sprague RL. Hyperactivity. In: *Symptoms of Psychopathology*, Costello GE (Ed.). New York: John Wiley & Sons, 1970.

CHAPTER 15

Specific Developmental Disorders (Learning Disabilities) of Childhood and Adolescence

Specific developmental disorders, more commonly referred to as learning disabilities, involve problems in reading, arithmetic, handwriting and/or language development that are not due to an intellectual defect, to an organic cause (blindness, deafness), or to other personality or environmental circumstances (see learning problems in Chapter 13). Children with learning disabilities, who are of at least average ability, tend to have difficulty in one area while achieving normally or above average in others. (Children with delayed language development may also do poorly in reading and arithmetic, however.) Learning disabilities tend to be identified in school when the child is having difficulty mastering specific learning tasks; they are usually not associated with psychopathology, except as a secondary consequence of the learning problem.

The functions of the health professional most often are those of ruling out organic causes for the learning problems and providing assistance in obtaining specialized services for the child. Therefore, it is important to be generally knowledgeable about these problems as a counselor to the parents, as a referral agent for specialist evaluations, and sometimes as an advocate for the child to obtain an appropriate educational program. Since children with learning disabilities usually suffer from a low self-image, it is important to help parents and others working with the child to learn to relate to the child's strengths, which are present in learning-disabled children. (In contrast, those who are moderately retarded have low functioning in all intellectual areas.)

Most characteristic of learning-disabled children is an inconsistency in their performance, whether on objective tests, in the classroom, or at home. Adults, peers, and the children themselves sense their innate intelligence. Their

155

failure to perform adequately in an area of weakness is often labeled as a "failure to try," "laziness," or "stupidity." The child does not understand his weakness, as a blind or deaf child would, nor do his peers or adults. Everyone knows that the child's performance does not meet expectations and a sense of failure becomes paramount. Once this assault on the self-image takes hold, secondary emotional and behavioral problems, such as acting out and disciplinary problems, school failure, dropout, delinquency, and depressed mood or passive withdrawal tend to occur.

Management by parents, teachers, physicians, and other professionals should include such statements as: "You are intelligent but you have a blind spot in this area." For a child whose strength is auditory, "You remember well what you hear, so say it to yourself several times"; "Take time to form your letters or correct yourself"; "Ask questions if you don't understand"; "Ask to hear it, if you cannot read it."

Positive statements that are realistic should be made: "You remember very well what you see, so write down what you hear"; "Since you do not easily remember well what I tell you, I will write it down for you because you remember what you see."

Four types of developmental disorders (reading, arithmetic, language, and articulation) are presented in this chapter. Although these disorders are quite common and increased professional attention has been devoted to them in recent years, both precise diagnosis and specific forms of intervention are still in the process of development. These disorders require referral to a specialist to make a diagnosis and further referral for intervention if a diagnosis of learning disability is confirmed; for that reason, flow charts are not provided here. The health provider's role in the diagnostic process is to rule out visual, auditory, neurological, and other organic deficits. Information is offered in the clinical management sections for each disorder to direct the health professional to resources for the child, as well as helping him or her work with parents. If a diagnosis of learning disabilities is not made in the specialist's evaluations, then other bases for the child's learning problems need to be explored. If mental retardation is the cause, this should be conveyed to the health professional in the psychologist's test report. If ability is normal, see the section on Learning Problems in Chapter 13 for other factors which may contribute to problems with school achievement.

DEVELOPMENTAL READING DISORDER

Clinical Picture

Reading disabilities are found in 3%–15% of school-age children, at a somewhat higher frequency among boys. Predisposing factors are not fully known, but children with a history of prenatal and perinatal difficulties have a greater tendency to show reading problems. Other possible causes include developmental lag, malnutrition and inadequate development of cerebral dominance. Frequently, there is cross-lateral or mixed dominance (e.g., a child may be right-handed and left-footed). There is some evidence of inherited tendencies for learning disabilities.

The kinds of reading problems presented by such children are quite varied. The better-known problems involve letter reversals such as confusing b, d, p, and q. Numerals such as 6 and 9 may also be reversed. Letters in words may be reversed at the end or in the middle. For instance, "was" may be read as "saw." Some learning-disabled children have difficulty recalling the names of printed words and are likely to have a weak sense of sentence structure. Once they develop basic reading skills, further problems with comprehension may also occur, due to the difficulty in reading rather than as a factor of intelligence. Poor visual memory will affect comprehension. Many children with reading disorders also have problems with spelling and with handwriting.

Ultimately, all tasks associated with the presented word become a source of anxiety, and efforts to avoid these activities are observed. Identification of these children can occur as early as kindergarten or first grade. The lack of readiness to read is often initially evident in the classroom in an inability to sit still and to work alone. Without special help, the child picks up minimal skills in the early grades, but is likely to be in serious academic trouble by third grade.

Diagnosis

According to DSM-III criteria, a developmental reading disorder is identified by performance on individualized tests showing reading skills that are significantly below the expected level, considering the child's education, chronological age, and intelligence (based on an individually administered IQ test). In this and all other learning disorders, "spiking," or an uneven profile of intellectual abilities is characteristic.

Following a medical assessment to determine that gross visual and auditory problems are not present, the next step is referral for a psychological assessment. The diagnostic battery should include an individual intelligence test, such as the Wechsler; an individual reading test, such as Slosson; and as other design-copying tests, such as the Bender-Gestalt, to assess the child's ability to reproduce spatial relationships.

Clinical Management

After the psychological evaluation, a diagnosis is likely to be communicated back to the health professional or to school personnel. If resources are available within the school system, the child may be assigned to individual or group tutoring by a special education teacher, in addition to regular classroom instruction. Depending on the differential diagnosis and age grouping, the special education teacher will provide various educational approaches, such as a linguistic approach to language, exercises for fine motor coordination, and graduated exercises for auditory memory span. In school systems without special education resources, the health professional may be able to locate resources in the community that provide special education tutoring (such as special education teachers who offer tutoring on an individual or group basis or special schools for learning-disabled children). Since reading disorders may coexist with other disorders, such as conduct disorders and hyperactivity, the health professional may consider referral to a mental health specialist for assistance with associated problems. Since damage to the child's self-image through repeated failures is a major concern, behavioral management techniques that recognize and reinforce real achievements and the child's strengths are essential. If the child remembers what he or she hears, then teach and communicate through that modality to the extent possible. For example, such children learn well with tape recorders. If visual memory is stronger, work with pictures, films, outlines, charts, etc. A major principle in working with learning-disabled children is to reduce barriers and demands for learning in the areas of weakness.

DEVELOPMENTAL ARITHMETIC DISORDER

Clinical Picture

Developmental arithmetic disorder may be found in upwards to 6% of school-age children. Certain abilities have been identified as essential to learning mathematics: general intelligence; spatial ability (seeing objects in relationship to others); verbal ability (vocabulary and comprehension); and approach to problem-solving (beginning logic). Weaknesses in any of these areas may show up in poor performance in arithmetic. While the mathematic tasks of the first few grades may be mastered by rote memory or memorization (even adding and subtracting on fingers and toes), as soon as the tasks require concepts of up and down, right and left, size relationships, and using multiple operations in a single problem, mastery of mathematics becomes problematic for children disabled in this area. Behavioral characteristics such as impulsivity and motor inhibition add to the child's problems and are seen in poorly constructed numerals and illegible characters. Although the course of this disorder cannot be described with any certainty, it generally seems to be chronic, extending into adolescence and beyond. Complications do not seem to involve conduct disorder as often as with children who have a reading disorder, but the poor school performance of affected children may result in low self-esteem. Once again, an uneven or "spiked profile" (a pattern of very strong and very weak areas of functioning) is seen in test results.

Diagnosis

The diagnosis of arithmetic disorder is based on significantly lower arithmetic achievement in contrast to what might be expected from the child's schooling, chronological age, and mental age. Diagnostic assessment, similar to that for reading disorder, involves referral for psychological testing and, at a minimum, would include an individually administered intelligence test and a test of arithmetic skills. The extent of the arithmetic problem and specific types of difficulty should be identified in this evaluation.

Clinical Management

Following psychological testing, findings would be reported back to the health professional and/or to school personnel. Many school systems offer individual or small-group teaching by a teacher with training in mathematics and special education. This resource varies from motor teaching (tracing numbers in sand) to more elaborate logic and strategy-type games. When specialized teaching is not available within the school system, the health professional, in concert with school personnel, may be able to identify tutoring resources in the community. Follow-up health care should include attention to the child's psychological and social adjustment and referral to a mental health specialist if the child manifests serious frustration with his or her school experiences and makes statements like "I am stupid" or "I am dumb." Once again, efforts should be made to identify the child's strengths and to encourage compensatory mechanisms, including the use of calculators and computers. Parents and teachers should be encouraged to identify the mode (i.e., auditory, visual, kinesthetic) in which the child learns best and to use it in whatever way possible. Frequently, the child will quite accurately answer the question: "Do you learn best by hearing, seeing, or watching/doing?" The health professional might say, "I will teach you how to use my stethoscope. Do you want me to tell you, show you, or let you read about how to do it?"

DEVELOPING LANGUAGE DISORDER

Clinical Picture

Children who are impaired in the development of language are likely to evidence delayed development in other important areas, including thought processes, play, and social and emotional functioning. Since language skills are necessary for reading, the language-delayed child almost always manifests learning problems in school.

Language disorders of two types are seen. The more common and less severe *expressive* type involves delayed speech that is not explained by general mental retardation or hearing impairment. Such children understand what is said to them, but have difficulty in verbal expression of thoughts and feelings. The *receptive* type, seen in less than 1% of children, involves impairment in both language production and in understanding what is communicated. A delay in spoken language is quite apparent by 18 months when even simple words such as "Mama" or "Dada" are not spoken. The desire to communicate is usually evident in eye contact between the child and mother when playing games like peekaboo. Once the child begins to speak, his or her language problem becomes apparent, demonstrated by errors in articulation, omission of certain sounds or difficulty naming objects. Further language acquisition continues to proceed at a slow rate.

The prognosis for children with developmental language disorders is generally positive. Even untreated, the child with *expressive* problems will eventually acquire language skills. For the child with a receptive disorder (i.e., failure to process and comprehend what is heard), language will probably never become normal unless treatment is received. Other consequences of language problems include lowered achievement in school as well as social and emotional complications, which underscore the importance of treatment and early detection.

Diagnosis

Diagnostic criteria for developmental language disorder include: (1) failure to develop vocal expression or (2) failure to develop comprehension and vocal expression of language, in the absence of mental retardation, pervasive development disorder, hearing impairment, or trauma.

Evaluation by the health professional involves ruling out hard signs of visual, auditory, and neurological impairment. If there are no positive findings, then referral for psychological testing is indicated. The psychological evaluation would include intellectual testing (to rule out mental retardation) and language testing to assess receptive language (e.g., with the Peabody Picture Vocabulary Test) and to identify the extent of impairment. Children with language disorders are likely to score better on the performance subtests (tests of visual-motor perception, memory, and coordination) of an individual intelligence test like the Wechsler Intelligence Scale for Children than on the verbal subtests which require language skills. Nevertheless, variation in verbal subtest scores is expected unless the child is retarded.

Clinical Management

Following testing, or when a diagnosis of language disorder is communicated to the health professional or school personnel, a referral for language therapy should be made as soon as possible. For the child with an expressive disorder (difficulty communicating as primary problem), therapeutic intervention will focus on vocabulary development, sentence construction and speech. Extra time should be given for the child with a receptive disorder to respond (understanding language is the primary problem). The child with a receptive disorder will require a program to develop auditory memory, auditory perception, and language comprehension. Again, extra time should be given for "processing," and the child should be spoken to slowly, in short, uncomplicated sentences. He or she should be asked to repeat what was said. No more than 2-3 instructions should be given at a time. Even if the child receives language therapy, the health professional will want to follow his or her progress and to watch for signs of associated psychological problems such as poor self-image. Parents and teachers should again be encouraged to reward successes and identify strengths. Visual memory may compensate for some of the child's language problems.

DEVELOPMENTAL ARTICULATION DISORDER

Clinical Picture

Developmental articulation disorder is a speech disorder that occurs with normal language development. Problems range from difficulty pronouncing a single sound to speech that is totally unintelligible. This disorder is a frequently seen problem in preschool and school-age children. The milder forms often disappear spontaneously, while the more severe forms may require years of treatment. As with the other types of learning disorders (except arithmetic) it is found more frequently in boys than in girls and is commonly thought to be caused by a maturational delay in the neurological processes necessary for clear speech. Clinical features involve omission, substitution, or distortion of consonant sounds. Examples of the preceding include: "bu" for "blue" (omission); "wabbit" for "rabbit" (substitution); and "putty" for "pretty" (distortion). For children who do not recover by age 9, speech therapy is indicated. However, for younger children who are seriously unintelligible, speech therapy is recommended at a younger age.

Diagnosis

The DSM-III diagnostic criteria for developmental articulation disorder include failure to develop consistent articulation of speech sounds such as r, sh, th, f, z, l, or ch, when this is not due to developmental language disorder (see preceding section of this chapter), mental retardation, or pervasive developmental disorder. Since these sounds are those acquired later and most children experience some difficulty in learning them, caution in assigning a diagnosis in the preschool years is appropriate.

For the health professional, audiometric, neurological, and medical examinations are necessary to rule out a physical basis. Since no characteristic pattern of responding to psychological tests has been found, referral for psychological testing is usually not necessary (assuming that the health professional can rule out mental retardation).

CLINICAL MANAGEMENT

Indications for speech therapy include any one of the following three situations: (1) problem with general intelligibility of speech at three years of age; (2) the child appears upset about his articulation difficulty; (3) continued problems with articulation beyond age 8. The health professional will want to assess the progress of the child through regular health visits. Parents and teachers should speak clearly themselves, acknowledge when they cannot understand the child, and ask for repetition. Giving positive reinforcement and encouragement to the child is important, as well as using all other modes of communication, (e.g., pointing, drawing).

REFERENCES

Jenkins RL. *Behavior Disorders of Childhood and Adolescence*. Springfield, Ill.: Charles C Thomas, 1973.

Rutter M, Martin JA. *The Child with Delayed Speech*. Philadelphia: J. B. Lippincott, 1972.

Sapir SG, Nitzburg AC. *Children with Learning Problems*. New York: Brunner/ Mazel, 1973.

CHAPTER 16

Conduct Disorders

The major characteristic of conduct disorders is a repetitive and persistent pattern of antisocial behavior that violates either the basic rights of others or major age-appropriate societal norms. Children with this disorder are constantly engaged in rule-breaking behavior that is more serious than the usual pranks of childhood or adolescence. The severity and frequency of these abnormal behaviors distinguishes these children from others, who may be considered stubborn or difficult.

Conduct disorders are common, especially in boys. Precise prevalence figures are not available. Some general population surveys have suggested that 5% to 15% of all children show conduct problems, although not necessarily ones that are serious enough to merit a diagnosis. Growing up under conditions of poverty, accompanied by family disorganization or separation, seems to be related to the occurrence of conduct disturbances. Behavioral deviations may also be due to a poor fit between a child's temperament and emotional needs and his or her parents' attitudes and practices. For example, a child may be very active and demanding, while the parents may expect the child to be calm and to move at their pace. Further, failure to develop a capacity for affection and trust in early attachments may be tied to later problems in developing relationships and in social behavior.

CLINICAL PICTURE

Characteristic behaviors of children with conduct disorder include stealing, fighting, destructive behavior (such as fire-setting), lying, and truancy. Stealing is the most usual presenting problem. These children frequently come to the attention of school or court authorities as a result of such behavior problems.

Behavioral problems are likely to occur at home, in school, and in the community, since such children tend to be in constant conflict with the world around them. Low academic achievement is common. Relationships with others, including peers, are generally not close, due in part to the low tolerance for frustration of children with conduct disorders and their tendency to blame others for difficulties. Low self-esteem is also observed, often masked by a tough exterior front.

The onset of conduct disorders varies from mid-childhood to adolescence. For about a third of these children, problems continue into adulthood in the form of Antisocial Personality Disorder. The long-range prognosis is related to the severity of behavioral problems, with the milder forms showing improvement over time.

DIAGNOSIS

The diagnostic process is based on the examination of three major groups of behaviors: aggressive conduct; nonaggressive conduct of a socially unacceptable nature; and capacity for social attachment. The fact that children differ with respect to aggressive versus nonaggressive patterns and in their ability to form social attachments has important implications for management. The Questionnaire for Conduct Disorders (page 164) can be administered to the parent or guardian to determine whether the diagnosis of Conduct Disorder should be made.

QUESTIONNAIRE FOR CONDUCT DISORDERS*

Has the child presented the following behavioral problems over the course of the past six months?

	YES	NO
1. Physical violence against persons or property (excluding those in defense of others or self), e.g., vandalism, fire-setting, mugging, assault?	——	—
2. Thefts involving confrontation with a victim (e.g., purse-snatching, armed robbery)?	——	—

---

*Adapted from DSM-III.

YES   NO

3. Chronic violation of a variety of important rules
   at home or school (e.g., persistent skipping of
   school or drug abuse)?   —— —
4. Repeated running away from home overnight?   —— —
5. Persistent lying, in and out of home?   —— —
6. Stealing that does not include confronting a victim? —— —

If one or more of the above items has occurred repeatedly over a six-month period, the diagnosis of Conduct Disorder is likely. When this disorder occurs along with hyperactivity or other developmental disorders, both diagnoses should be made.

Before considering a plan for intervention, it is also necessary to assess the extent of social attachment between the child or adolescent and others, as this has implications for change based on a relationship-oriented therapeutic approach. Ask the parent or guardian the following about his or her child:

YES   NO

1. Has the child at least one peer-group friendship that has
   lasted over six months?   —— —
2. Will the child help others even when no immediate benefit is expected?   —— —
3. Does the child seem to feel guilt or remorse appropriately—not just when caught?   —— —
4. Does the child tend not to blame or tell on companions? —— —
5. Does the child appear concerned about the welfare of
   friends or companions?   —— —

A child for whom none of the items of the last group of statements is true presents a different picture clinically than the child for whom two or more of the preceding statements are characteristic. Positive responses indicate that the child places some value on relationships with others and is likely to respond more quickly to psychotherapeutic intervention.

CLINICAL MANAGEMENT

The child with a true conduct disorder is one of the most difficult types of children for health professionals to work with. The behaviors, if well established, are slow to change. Family members often feel frustrated in their efforts to make the child's behavior more socially acceptable. They may feel embarrassed about being called into conferences at school or with the police or courts regarding their child's behavior problems. Ultimately, many parents

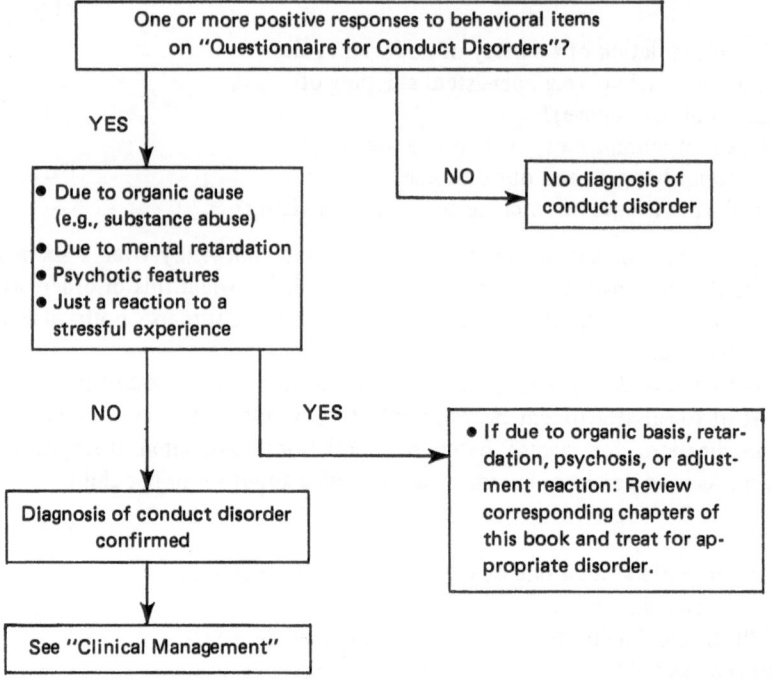

Figure 16.1. Conduct disorders of childhood, diagnostic flow chart

feel anger toward the child, which may become directed toward the helping professional.

The child who engages in antisocial behavior but has some ability to form trusting relationships is less difficult to work with than the child who does not invest feelings in relationships with others. Working with the latter type of children may not be very gratifying for the health professional who, after extensive efforts to help, may find out, for example, that he or she has been lied to repeatedly. The health professional needs to anticipate that the course of working with the child and his or her family may be a rugged one, in order to prevent becoming disappointed or angry in the helping process. Firmness and impartiality with the child and family are necessary, but difficult to maintain.

A major contribution that the health professional can make is to identify and intervene in the early stages of the development of problematic behavior. This can occur through inquiring systematically about the child's social adjustment during regular health-maintenance visits. For example, the health professional can ask how the child gets along with peers in the neighborhood or with his or her teachers at school.

The initial approaches to clinical management are similar, whether the conduct problems are at an early stage or a diagnosis of conduct disorder has been made. When the parents seek help for their child, they are likely to be upset and angry. Often the child's problematic behavior will have been brought to their attention by school or legal authorities. Initially, there may be a tendency to minimize the problem or to seek a medical explanation. The health professional can help to calm them down by reviewing the behaviors and events of concern and by providing them with an opportunity to talk about their feelings and worries. Since the parents' feelings of anger or frustration toward the child may have overshadowed positive feelings, encouraging feelings of acceptance and warmth toward the child is the next step, after accepting the parents' own feelings about the child. This may involve helping the parents to recall the child's strengths or positive attributes.

The next major step is to develop a plan to alter the child's behavior; this involves the selection of the behaviors to focus on first. If a child is skipping school, lying, stealing, and experimenting with drugs, it is not possible to work on all these problems with equal energy. While it is important to communicate to the child that changes in the preceding behaviors will be expected over time, setting a priority on one or two is sufficient initially. Expectations need to be communicated clearly, along with a plan for supervising the child's behavior and the consequences of violations. Children with conduct disorders are not likely to respond at all to severe punishment. Their "tough" exterior presentation communicates the message "you can't hurt me," and despite internal feelings of helplessness and self-hatred, the usual methods of punishment will not penetrate the surface. Punishment therefore needs to be tied directly to the behavior, e.g., doing chores for a neighbor to compensate for the value of an object stolen from the neighbor, or cleaning up a house after vandalizing it. The aim of punishment is to help the child experience the consequences of his unacceptable behavior. It also needs to be tied closely in time to the event of the unacceptable behavior.

While it is necessary to help parents communicate clearly and to respond consistently to unacceptable behavior, it is equally important to help them learn to give the child credit for appropriate behavior. Since children with conduct disorders tend to be "in trouble" so much of the time, they get to the point of never expecting a positive word. Positive recognition for desirable behavior offers a stronger approach to achieving change in behavior than does punishment or attribution of guilt for negative behavior.

Following the initial evaluation, coordination with school or other personnel directly concerned about the child's behavior should be initiated so that efforts to alter the child's behavior are consistent. Since other agencies may be working with the child, it is essential that a key coordinating professional be identified. Because of the child's ability to successfully manipulate others, it is essential that one professional be designated as the primary provider. This is likely to be the person or agency most closely associated with the problem be-

Once the diagnosis is confirmed,
spend about two months in the following steps:

1. Meet several times with parents or family to:

   a. review problematic behaviors (including events that
      precede and follow) and parents' feelings about child;
   b. encourage acceptance and communication of warmth toward
      child;
   c. establish expectations of behavioral changes and be sure they
      are clearly communicated to the child;
   d. develop a plan for responding to violations, including
      any punishment that would be a consequence;
   e. work with parents on providing structure in the child's
      daily life;
   f. also develop a way to recognize and reward appropriate
      behavior;
   g. Help parents understand that behavioral change will not
      occur very quickly and that their role will not be a
      rewarding one initially. Progress is likely to come
      more slowly if the child has not formed social attach-
      ments to peers or adults.

2. Coordinate efforts with school or court personnel involved
   with the child.
3. Schedule two follow-up sessions, two weeks apart, to review
   progress and further issues; if improvement has been observed,
   schedule follow-up in one month.

If improvement in the child's behavior is minimal:

4. Consider referral to a mental health specialist. Reality or behaviorally oriented group therapy or family treatment are possible
   options.
5. Consider placement in a residential school, which becomes necessary for some children.
6. Do not prescribe medication or refer for individual psychotherapy.

Figure 16.2.   Conduct disorders of childhood, management flow chart

haviors (e.g., for stealing, it may be the court worker; for skipping school, the
school counselor; for fighting with siblings at home, the health professional).

   Work with the parents directed toward venting feelings, establishing behavioral expectations and consequences for violating them, and recognizing

positive behavior is likely to occupy two to four sessions. Several follow-up appointments could be scheduled at about two-week intervals to review progress and discuss any further problems.

Problems that may come up in follow-up sessions include worsening of behavior or conflict between parents about differences in handling the child's misbehavior. An increase in unacceptable behavior on the part of the child is not unusual when new procedures for handling a child's behavior are introduced. The child will test the seriousness of the parents' intentions. If the parents can persist, the child will begin to realize that they are serious, and the health professional can provide some reassurance in this vein. In the event that parents are in conflict about behavioral expectations or consequences, helping them to clarify the source of the disagreement is a first step. Do they differ in how they understand the plan or do they usually disagree on what will be effective with their child. A *consistent* approach toward the child is essential. If the problem is related to the plan itself, the health professional can probably help the parents clarify their differences and suggest revisions to the plan. However, if long-term conflict between the parents becomes apparent, then referral for family counseling or family therapy may be advisable. Many children with conduct disorders grow up in families disrupted by dissent, separation, or divorce, where help from a mental health specialist may be needed for the parents as much as for the child.

If over a two-month period, after several planning sessions and several follow-up visits, progress in the child's behavior has been reported, a further visit might be scheduled for the following month. If, instead, the child's behavioral problems persist or worsen, then serious consideration should be given to referral to a mental health specialist.

The mental health specialist is likely to select among several treatment approaches for conduct disorders. Children with some ability to form relationships can usually benefit from behaviorally oriented group therapy. Family therapy can be useful to examine interaction patterns between the child and family members and to help family members learn to avoid being manipulated by the child with a conduct disorder. Other recently tested therapeutic approaches, such as reality therapy, may help the child assume responsibility for his or her behavior through learning that there are consequences to unacceptable behavior. Individual psychotherapy and psychotropic medication are not recommended for children with conduct disorders.

For the child (or, more usually, the adolescent) who does not respond to any of the preceding approaches, temporary placement in an institutional setting such as a residential school may be required. When the behavior is out of control and dangerous to the individual or others, such a placement provides the structure and consistent limit-setting that restricts antisocial behavior while also providing intensive group-oriented therapy. Untreated, many of these children end up in correctional settings through a court order, which usually do not offer therapeutic services.

In conclusion, the health professional may have an opportunity to intervene constructively in conduct disorders at an early stage. Major concepts to help parents with are consistent discipline and structure, which may include such matters as regular bedtime and mealtimes or expecting the child to perform regular household duties. Also important is coordination with other professionals such as teachers to ensure that the behaviors being worked on at home are also attended to in school. If no positive changes result, referral of the child and family to mental health specialists is recommended. When highly antisocial and aggressive patterns of behavior are well established, immediate referral to a mental health service should be considered.

CHAPTER 17

Anxiety Disorders of Childhood

Anxiety in children may be described as intense and diffuse feelings of apprehension or impending disaster. Anxiety is experienced by children as an unpleasant sensation accompanied by restlessness, fatigue, and such visceral components as headaches, a "funny feeling" in the stomach, or heaviness in the
chest. In an acute anxiety attack, the sense of uneasiness is intensified and children may cling to parents, cry out in fear, and complain about physiological
symptoms (perspiration, fast heartbeat, and difficulty breathing). Such attacks,
which tend to have a brief duration, are very frightening to the child and to
those around her or him.

CLINICAL PICTURE

The types* of anxiety manifested by children include:

Performance Anxiety

Also known as *Overanxious disorder*, it is seen in children who fear failure
and feel incompetent, particularly in school, although they may even have a history of outstanding achievement.

Fear of loss, abandonment or separation

This type of anxiety is seen in children who have difficulty separating from
parents beyond a time when it is developmentally appropriate. It is known as
separation anxiety and usually is manifested as school phobia.

---

*These terms and their definitions are adapted from DSM-111.

Social Anxiety

This is exhibited by shy children, who have a sense of embarrassment and fear of humiliation and ridicule in new social situations.

Phobias

These are seen in children as fixed fears that persist beyond the time when they are commonly experienced. (For preschool children to fear animals, storms, darkness, doctors, strange persons, and unfamiliar situations is common, and therefore is not considered a phobia, as it might be in an older child.)

This chapter focuses on performance anxiety (overanxious disorder), and on separation anxiety disorder (the fear of loss or abandonment), because they are the most common types of anxiety disorders in children. Phobias, with the exception of school phobia, are not addressed in this chapter. Discomfort with new social situations and strangers, known in DSM-III as Avoidant Disorder of Childhood or Adolescence, is thought to be relatively uncommon and is useful primarily to distinguish such children from those with more severe withdrawal, who generally show little interest in social situations of any kind.

PERFORMANCE ANXIETY (OVERANXIOUS DISORDER)

Overanxious children present with excessive worrying and fearful behavior that is not focused on a specific situation or event. The overanxious disorder may appear gradually or suddenly and may be incapacitating to the extent that the child cannot meet basic expectations at home and in school. This disorder is more likely to occur among children from upper socioeconomic groups, in which a superior level of achievement is expected.

Differential Diagnosis

Some of the symptoms, particularly fearfulness, somatic complaints, and difficulty falling asleep, are also seen in separation anxiety. However, the situations associated with discomfort are clearly differentiated. The overanxious child is generally fearful about his ability to perform in social or school situations, while discomfort in the child with separation anxiety occurs when anticipating or experiencing separation from parents and familiar situations.

Since some level of anxiety is present in most childhood developmental and other disorders, the possibility that anxiety is secondary to another disorder should be carefully considered. For example, a learning-disabled child may be constantly anxious due to his inability to master academic tasks. Anxiety symptoms may also be caused by clinical or undiagnosed physical conditions (e.g., anemia, hypoglycemia, poor nutrition, poor vision, poor hearing), which need to be explored. Other sources of stress in the child's environment (e.g., conflict between the child's parents) also need to be assessed carefully during evaluation.

DIAGNOSIS

The Questionnaire* for the Diagnosis of Performance Anxiety can be given to the parents or guardian to determine the diagnosis of performance anxiety.

QUESTIONNAIRE FOR THE DIAGNOSIS OF PERFORMANCE ANXIETY (OVERANXIOUS DISORDER)

Has the child experienced any of the following problems during the past six months?

	YES	NO
1. Unrealistic worry about future events?	—	—
2. Excessive worry about the acceptability of his or her behavior?	—	—
3. An exaggerated concern that he or she is not competent in a variety of areas (e.g., academic, athletic, social)?	—	—
4. Need for constant reassurance about worries?	—	—
5. Somatic complaints such as headaches or stomachaches, for which no physical basis can be established?	—	—
6. Marked feelings of self-consciousness?	—	—

If four or more of the above items are present and they have persisted for at least six months, the diagnosis of performance anxiety is likely if there is no evidence of separation anxiety, phobia, or other disorder.

CLINICAL MANAGEMENT

The management of an acute anxiety attack may be the first task presented to the health professional. After ruling out a physical cause, the health professional will usually be able to obtain a fairly rapid response through reassuring

---

*Adapted from DSM-III.

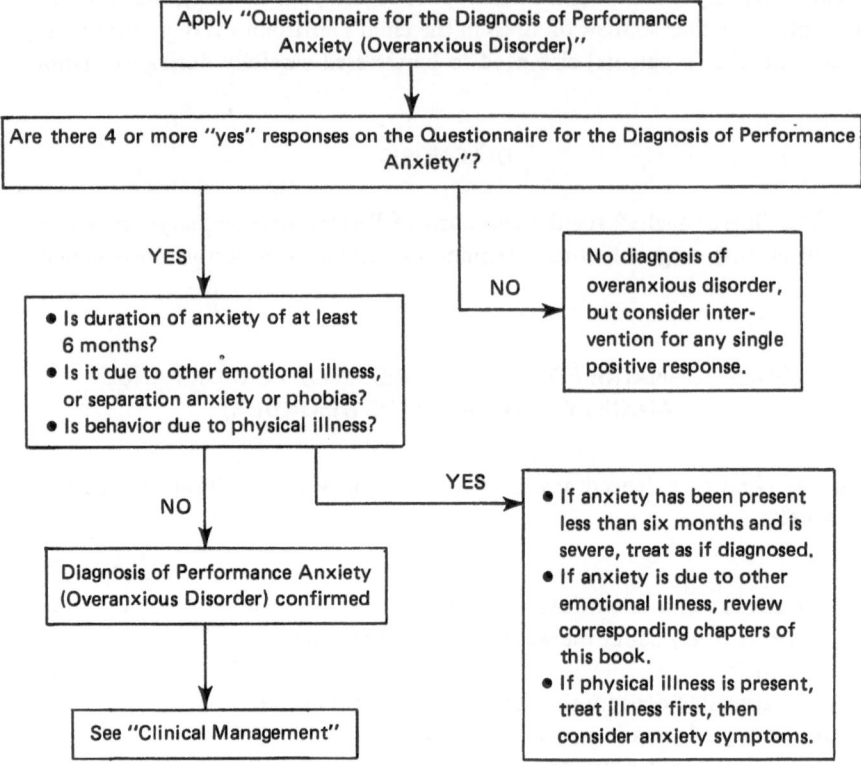

Figure 17.1. Performance anxiety (overanxious disorder) of childhood, diagnostic flow chart

words and a calm approach. The child should be told that he or she will feel better very soon and that the health professional understands what he or she is feeling. Parents can learn from the health professional to apply the same approach at home.

Some environmental manipulation to reduce stress on the child may be necessary initially. This may include: (1) communicating reduced achievement expectations (e.g., parents or teachers may tell the child that it is not necessary at this time to make honor roll grades); (2) fostering successful experiences in areas in which the child is fearful and giving recognition for approaching frightening tasks; parents may need help in identifying and rewarding very small steps

Spend 6–8 weeks in the following steps:

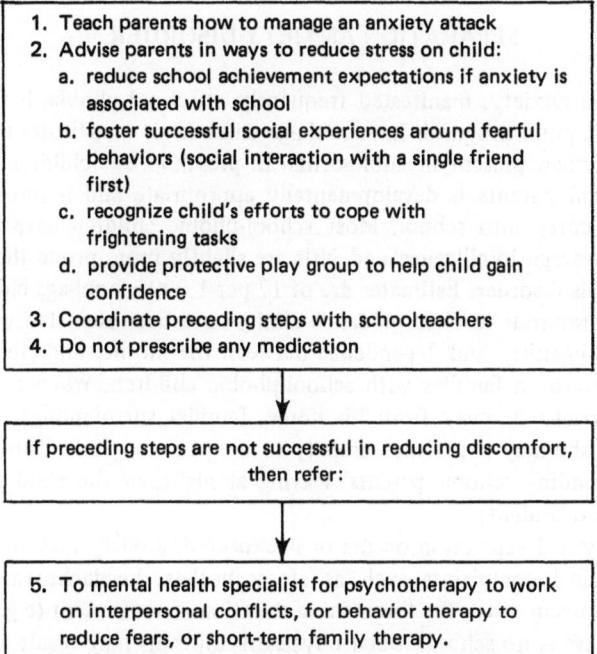

1. Teach parents how to manage an anxiety attack
2. Advise parents in ways to reduce stress on child:
   a. reduce school achievement expectations if anxiety is associated with school
   b. foster successful social experiences around fearful behaviors (social interaction with a single friend first)
   c. recognize child's efforts to cope with frightening tasks
   d. provide protective play group to help child gain confidence
3. Coordinate preceding steps with schoolteachers
4. Do not prescribe any medication

If preceding steps are not successful in reducing discomfort, then refer:

5. To mental health specialist for psychotherapy to work on interpersonal conflicts, for behavior therapy to reduce fears, or short-term family therapy.

Figure 17.2. Performance anxiety (overanxious disorder) management flow chart (diagnosis confirmed)

made by the child; (3) providing protective small-group activities led by an adult, which can be used to foster interaction between a child and his peers. The health professional can advise parents about such approaches, but may also need to communicate directly with school personnel regarding application of the preceding approaches to management of the child's fears in school.

After a trial of several months, if the preceding steps have not successfully altered the child's discomfort in school or social situations, referral for more intensive mental health services by specialists may be recommended to the parents. Individual psychotherapy may be indicated when there is conflict in the child's relationships. Also, behavioral approaches such as relaxation and desensitization are useful to reduce fears in situations such as test-taking. Short-term family therapy is usually helpful in facilitating changes in patterns of interaction that tend to perpetuate the anxiety of the child.

SEPARATION ANXIETY DISORDER

Separation anxiety, manifested frequently as school phobia, is fairly common and has a good prognosis in school-age children; it constitutes a more serious problem when present in adolescents. In preschool-age children, difficulty separating from parents is developmentally appropriate and is most likely to show up on entry into school. Most school-phobic children have average or higher than average intelligence and girls are slightly more prone than boys to suffer from this disorder. Estimates are of 17 per 1,000 school-age children, and 2% to 8% of referrals to child guidance clinics have been reported with school phobia. Both hostility and dependence between the mother and child is a predominant pattern in families with school-phobic children. When a child with separation anxiety is away from his home, familiar surroundings or parental figures, he or she may experience anxiety to the point of panic. This may interfere with attending school, parents' leaving at night, or the child going to a friend's house overnight.

When physical separation occurs or is expected, anxiety may be expressed through physical complaints such as stomachaches, headaches and nausea, which do not occur when the threatening situation is not present (e.g., on weekends when there is no school). Such physical symptoms may result in frequent visits to the doctor. Preoccupation with fear of animals, monsters, or situations seen as presenting danger to the family are also common. Difficulty falling asleep, fear of the dark, trying to sleep in their parents' bed, and nightmares expressing morbid fears are ways of expressing fears and contribute to difficult evenings for the child and the family.

Differential Diagnosis

Separation anxiety is clearly an excessive reaction to separation from parents or other important figures in the child's life, in contrast to performance anxiety. Anxiety about separation may be a factor in more severe mental disorders of children, but the anxiety is clearly associated with these conditions (e.g., depression). When a child meets diagnostic criteria for both major depression and separation anxiety disorder, both diagnoses should be made. Separation anxiety must also be differentiated from truancy (avoidance of school attendance for other activities, which are also usually away from the home), realistic fear of a threatening situation in school, and from school avoidance because of learning difficulties.

DIAGNOSIS

The Questionnaire for the Diagnosis of Separation Anxiety* can be given to the parents or guardians of the child to determine the diagnosis of separation anxiety. Particular attention should be given to the child's recent school attendance history.

QUESTIONNAIRE FOR THE DIAGNOSIS OF SEPARATION ANXIETY

Has the child experienced any of the following problems during the last six months?

	YES	NO
1. Unrealistic worry that something serious would happen to either parents or child to separate them?	——	—
2. Persistent refusal or hesitance to go to school in order to remain home with parent? If yes, how often?——	——	—
3. Persistent reluctance to go to sleep without a parent present, persistent reluctance to sleep away from home?	——	—
4. Fear of being alone at home or in a separate room from parent?	——	—
5. Repeated nightmares about separation (e.g., about getting lost in the woods)?	——	—
6. Symptoms like headaches or stomachaches on school days?	——	—
7. Excessive distress when parents leave the child (applicable to children over six)?	——	—
8. Sadness, worry, and difficulty playing or concentrating when not with a parent?	——	—

If four or more of the above items are answered "yes" and they have persisted for at least six months, the diagnosis of separation anxiety is likely if there is no evidence of performance anxiety, phobia, or other disorder. The health professional should be able to identify this disorder long before six months have elapsed.

CLINICAL MANAGEMENT

Separation anxiety is frequently improved without treatment by mental health professionals. In the case of recent onset, the health professional should assess life stress affecting the child, such as the death of a loved person or the

---

*Adapted from DSM–III.

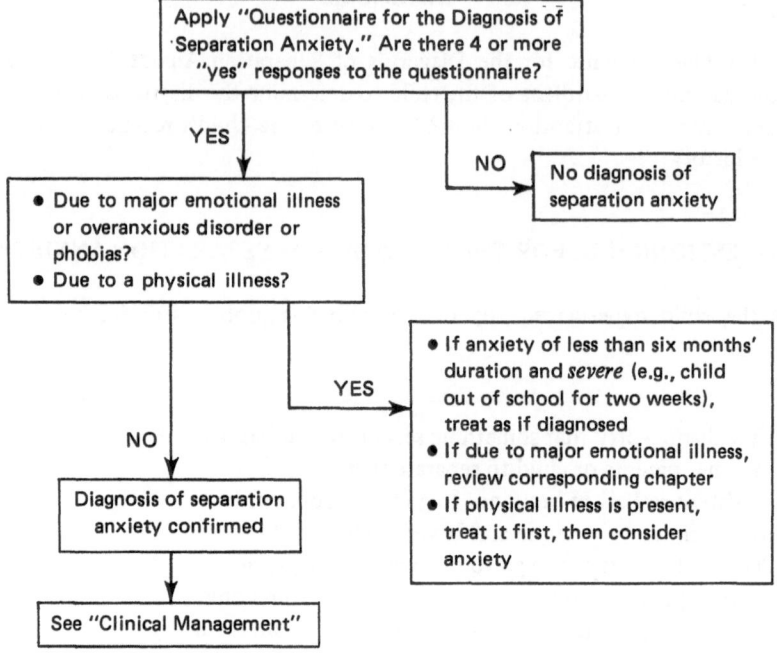

Figure 17.3. Separation anxiety, diagnostic flow chart

loss of valued objects; an illness of the child or relative; or a major environmental change. If the traumatic event occurred recently, then it may be sufficient for the health professional to give support and reassurance that the event is not likely to recur, with instructions for the parent to follow through. This involves encouraging parents to help the child discuss his or her feelings about the uncomfortable or frightening event.

When separation anxiety is manifested in failure to attend school, the following steps are preliminary to planning the child's return to school:

1. Assess whether the parent(s) contributes to the child's staying at home through either a need for company or a fear that something harmful will happen to the child in school. Without full parental support for school attendance, further steps will not succeed.
2. After insuring that the child does not have a medical condition that contributed to staying at home, de-emphasize child's medical complaints by stating to both parent(s) and child that you think the child is able to attend school.

Spend 6 weeks in the following steps:

1. Assess life stress and, if problems seem to have been precipitated by a recent event, provide support and reassurance to parents and child.
2. Explore parental involvement in child's staying home and seek parental support for child's return to school.
3. After medical conditions are ruled out, de-emphasize the child's medical complaints with both parents and child.
4. Help parents reduce positive aspects of remaining at home, but do not foster guilt feelings in the parents or the child.
5. Plan child's return to school with parents and school personnel.
6. Remain firm about school attendance while communicating an understanding of the child's fears and the parents' concern about their child.

If the preceding steps do not result in regular school attendance and reduced anxiety:

7. Referral to a mental health specialist is necessary for intensive behavioral or other psychotherapeutic intervention.
8. As a general rule, do not prescribe any medication.

Figure 17.4. Separation anxiety, management flow chart

3. Help parents think through ways to reduce positive aspects of the child being home on school days (e.g., eliminating extra attention or special treats).
4. School counselors, nurses, principal, and assistant principals are key persons in facilitating the return of the child to school. Engage school personnel in planning the child's return to school. A conference between the teacher, parents and health professional can be used to explain to school personnel that although the child has some fears about leaving home and going to school, it is very important for him or her to do so (see the next item for specific steps). Sometimes the child needs to be placed in a special education classroom (small group, better structure) on a transitory basis before he or she is ready to return to the regular classroom.

A rapid return to school is critical!

The longer the child is out, the more difficult the return. Helping the child feel safe in school can be facilitated by careful planning. The health professional can assist parents in breaking this process down into small enough steps for the child to tolerate. Such steps might include the following: a parent(s) takes the child for a walk around the school on a weekend; a parent(s) takes the child into class when only the teacher is present, such as after school; a parent(s) stays in class briefly with the child when school is in session; a parent(s) remains in the building for a brief period of time when the child is in class.

Throughout the process of returning the child to school, the health professional must remain firm about school attendance and supportive when pain and fears are expressed. Special meetings with parents can be scheduled (possibly 15-minute sessions weekly) after the initial plan has been developed. It is important to help parents understand that the child's fear is related to leaving home, not a fear of school, but that the only way to get over it is to go to school. The parents also need to work intensively on their own conflicts and need to keep the child at home.

If after four weeks time the preceding steps have not resulted in regular school attendance, referral to a mental health specialist for more intensive intervention may be necessary.

CHAPTER 18

Childhood Disorders
with Physical Manifestations
(Enuresis, Encopresis, and Stuttering)

This chapter covers three problems of childhood: enuresis (wetting), encopresis (fecal soiling), and stuttering. In the past, these problems were thought to develop mainly from psychological conflicts and to be associated with other signs of psychopathology. Currently these problems are not viewed as symptomatic of major psychopathology, but are seen as benefiting from limited psychological intervention. Although most of the children who have enuresis, encopresis, or who stutter do not have associated mental disorders, effective management of such children and their parents is important in order to prevent damaging psychological consequences. Both enuresis and stuttering are quite common in young children and encopresis, although rare, is presented because of the difficulty in handling it. The diagnosis of these disorders is relatively simple, therefore a questionnaire is not required. Instructions regarding the diagnostic assessment are included.

ENURESIS

Enuresis is defined as the repetitive, inappropriate, and involuntary passage of urine in a child who does not have an organic condition that might account for it and who is beyond an age when control over this function is expected to have occurred. Enuresis is seen twice as frequently in boys than in girls, due possibly to the slower physiological maturation of boys. It is more of an issue during the cold seasons of year or when the child sleeps in a cold room. Most enuretic children wet only at night (about 80%); a much smaller group wets both at night and in the daytime (15%); and only about 5% wet in the daytime only. Those who wet only at night are less likely to have organic pathology than those who wet in the daytime or both during the day and at night.

Clinical Picture

Enuresis is more likely to stem from maturational or developmental factors than from psychodynamic ones. Psychological issues become important because of the social consequence of wetting and poor parental management, rather than as the cause of it. Difficult or inadequate toilet training may become associated with anxiety around toilet training and urinating. The usual clinical course of enuresis is spontaneous remission at ages 6 or 7 or in puberty. Enuresis should not be viewed as abnormal, particularly in boys, until after they are 5 years of age. There are several situations in which enuresis may be differentially responsive to treatment: (1) a strong family history of enuresis, particularly on the father's side, in which sleepwalking and sleeptalking are common; and (2) enuresis that occurs sometime after the child has been dry, associated with trouble separating from parents, or with depression.

Diagnosis

Enuresis is arbitrarily defined as involuntary wetting at least twice a month for children between the ages of 5 and 6 and once a month for older children. The disorder is considered primary enuresis if consistent dryness has never been achieved and secondary when a child has been dry for a year and begins wetting again. Secondary enuresis tends to occur following a critical event in the child's life such as the birth of a sibling or hospitalization for a medical condition. The diagnostic process should include the following types of assessments:

1. A thorough physical examination and urinalysis to rule out physical abnormalities or the presence of diseases such as diabetes, epilepsy, sickle cell anemia, internal parasites, infections, or a condition like mental retardation (see Chapter 19 on mental retardation).
2. Characteristics of the wetting pattern (e.g., frequency, association with recent events) and parental efforts made to achieve dryness (e.g., rewards, punishment, getting the child up at night, withholding liquids before bedtime).
3. Family or psychosocial factors such as conflict in the home, inadequate bathroom facilities, and sleeping habits which might contribute to the problem.
4. The possibility of an emotional disturbance such as anxiety (see Chapter 17, Anxiety Disorders of Childhood).

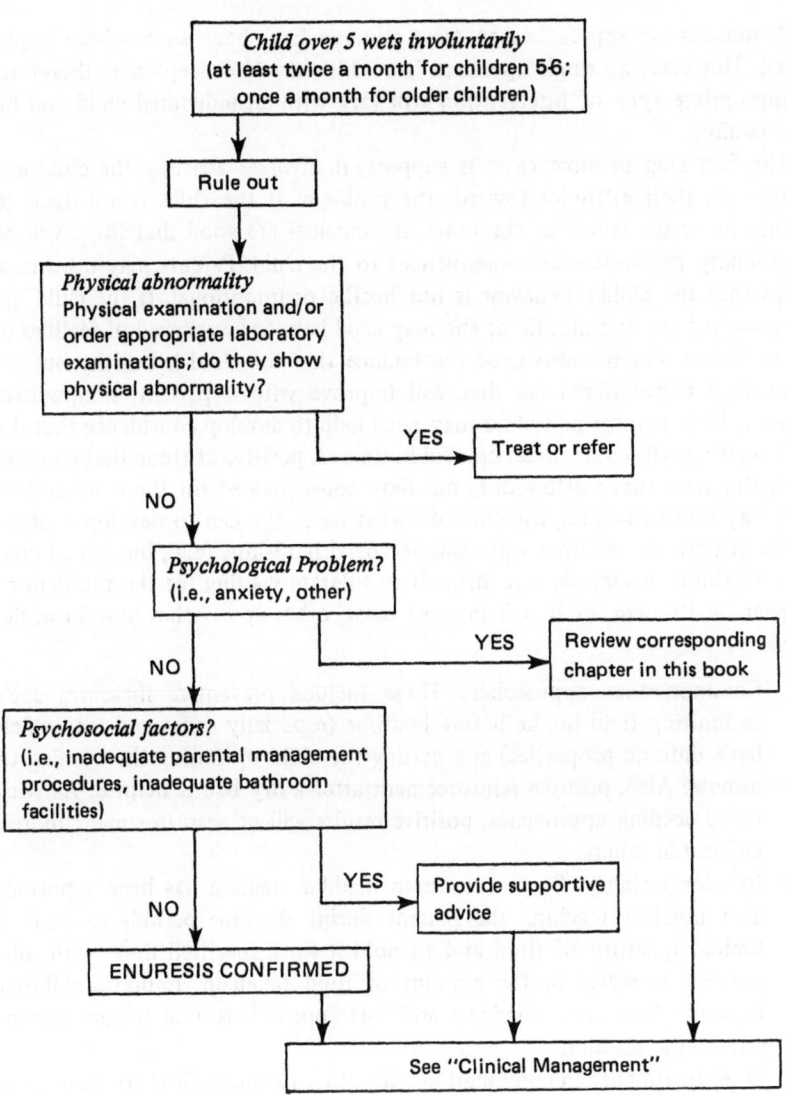

Figure 18.1.   Enuresis, diagnostic flow chart

Clinical Management

A number of approaches to treat enuresis have been successfully implemented. However, no single approach has achieved wide acceptance; therefore,
the appropriate type of intervention will vary with an individual child and his
or her family.

The first step in most cases is support; it involves assisting the child and
parents with their attitudes towards the problem. If the child is not made to
feel that he or she is bad or abnormal, the chances are good that there will be
no secondary psychological consequences to the child. Parents may need reassurance that the child's behavior is not hostile or intentional. If the child has
been punished for wetting, he or she may need help to be relieved of feelings of
guilt or shame. Parents also need reassurance that the child is healthy but experiencing a maturational lag that will improve with a patient, nonpunitive
approach. Both parents and child may need help to develop confidence that the
child's wetting will come under control in time. A positive attitude that communicates the view that wetting does not have consequences for the child will go
a long way toward helping the child do what he or she can to develop control.

For parents or children who—due to social hardships (e.g., burden of constantly washing sheets)—find it difficult to tolerate waiting for the problem to
disappear on its own, as it will in most cases, other approaches have been described:

1. Common-sense approaches: These include preventive measures such
   as limiting fluid intake before bedtime (especially sodas and tea, which
   have diuretic properties) and getting the child up during the evening to
   urinate. Also, positive reinforcement after a dry bed is helpful. As with
   the preceding approaches, positive results will be seen in some children
   and not in others.
2. Bladder training: Some success in bladder training has been reported.
   This involves teaching the patient during daytime periods to drink a
   limited quantity of fluid and to hold it for a specified time, with subsequent increases in the amount of fluid taken in. Enuretic children
   typically have small bladders and this approach is used to successively
   stretch the bladder.
3. Drug treatment: In combination with other methods, drug treatment has
   been found to be useful, particularly for brief periods of time. Imipramine can be prescribed in doses of 10–40 mg at bedtime for a 6–8 week
   trial and withdrawn over a 4-week period. Higher doses, of 25-75 mg,
   may be more effective than lower ones in older latency age children.
   Enuretic behavior is likely to recur following drug withdrawal. In addition, side effects such as restlessness, irritability, weight loss and gastrointestinal upsets should be anticipated.

Step 1: Support
  • Be supportive 1. to the child (wetting does not mean that the child
                      is bad);
                   2. to parents. (Explain that controlling wetting is a
                      maturational process that takes longer in some
                      children than in others.)
  • Reassure parents that behavior is not hostile or intentional
  • Relieve guilt feelings on the child's part
  • Advise parents NOT to punish child for wetting

Step 2: Suggest common-sense approach.
  • Limit fluid intake before bedtime
  • Get child up during the evening to go to the bathroom

Step 3: Explain bladder-training approach

Step 4: Suggest drug treatment
  • Imipramine, 10–40 mg at bedtime for 6–8-week trial; withdraw
    over 4-week period.

Step 5: With caution, consider using conditioning device (explain its
        mechanism)

Step 6: Anticipate relapses associated with overexertion and expect a brief
        duration.

Figure 18.2. Enuresis, management flow chart

4. A conditioning device: A pad placed on the bed is attached to a bell, wired such that the first drop of urine causes a bell to ring. The bell alerts the child to go to the bathroom, but it may also wake up other members of the family instead of the intended child. Because of the preceding complications, this approach is considered controversial.

The preceding approaches can be tried in any order, depending on the individual case. In resistant cases, referral for individual behavior modification techniques or individual and/or family therapy is indicated. In working with enuretic children, it is important to remember that following remission, relapses may occur. Relapses are usually associated with fatigue, hard play, or emotional conflicts, and parents need encouragement that such recurrences are likely to be of brief duration. Punishment is never justified.

ENCOPRESIS

Encopresis is defined as involuntary defecation at least once a month in inappropriate places and is not due to disease or deformity; it occurs beyond an age (around 4) where bowel control is physiologically possible and after toilet training should be completed. More recently, inappropriate voluntary defecation has been included in the definition of encopresis. Although seen rarely (1.5% of children), it is highly problematic for the child, the family, and the health professional since treatment results are frequently far from successful. Boys seem to be about five times more likely than girls to develop this problem.

Clinical Picture

Soiling is seen in very different types of children. In the mentally retarded, encopresis may be a function of the overall defect (particularly in the severely retarded child) and special approaches to toilet training may be required for the child with a lower level of ability. The child with attention deficit disorder or hyperactivity may soil because he/she fails to attend to such bodily functions and does not think about the need to locate the bathroom when he/she is outside playing a game. Other children soil as a result of parental failure to make any effort to train the child, while for another group the problem may be associated with harsh or punitive toilet training, of which the latter is related to the child's needs to accommodate his or her bodily functions to the needs of the parents. Finally, some children with other emotional problems soil sporadically as a reaction to psychological stress or to a specific threatening situation (e.g., being spoken to firmly by a parent or other authority figure). In many encopretic children, little contact with fathers has been described, while strong interaction with mothers is predominant.

Soiling with associated abdominal pain, constipation or fecal impactment demands medical assessment. In approximately one-fourth of the cases, constipation is associated with soiling.

In the course of this disorder, which usually disappears by adolescence, the child may suffer hostility within the family as well as alienation from peers and teachers. Frequently, a complaint from school is the stimulus that prompts the parent to take the child to the health professional. Further, many encopretic children do not know when they need to defecate, are unaware of the effect of their behavior on others and consequently do not understand others' reactions toward them.

Diagnosis

In the diagnostic process it is important to assess the following areas: (1) family climate (extent of conflict in the family); (2) practices used for bowel training (Was the child forced or threatened?); (3) the family's reaction to and management of the child's soiling; and (4) the child's self-perception (e.g., negative versus positive self-image). A diagnosis of functional encopresis is made when repeated voluntary or involuntary defecation occurs in inappropriate

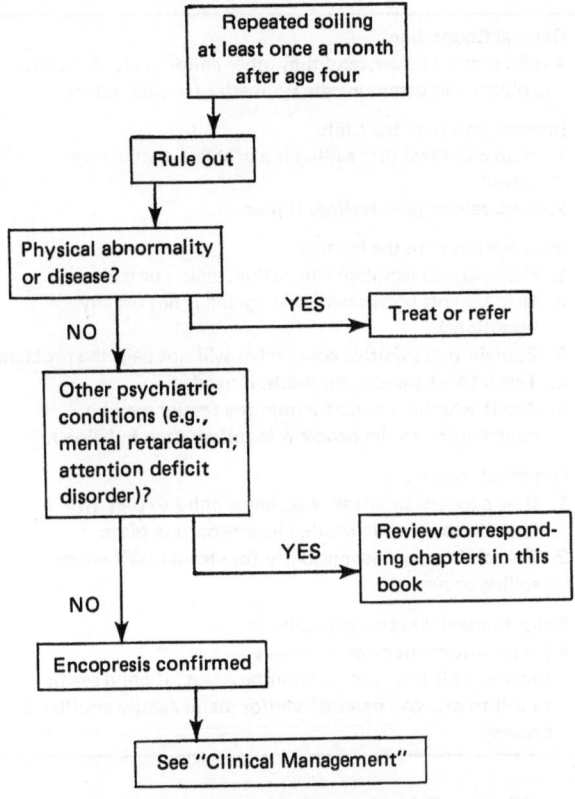

Figure 18.3. Encopresis, diagnostic flow chart

places at least once a month after the age of 4. It is important to rule out other physical disorders, such as Hirschsprung's disease (enlargement of the colon resulting from an obstruction) and to identify psychiatric conditions such as mental retardation and attention deficit disorder, which may be associated with encopresis.

Clinical Management

Once a diagnosis of encopresis is made, there are some general principles that apply to intervention and approaches that are specific to an individual child, which should be based on information obtained in the process of assessing the problem. General principles in the management of encopresis involve helping parents understand that there are others with the same problem, giving parents a

Step 1: General Counseling
- Help parents understand that other children also have this problem and communicate sympathy for their plight

Step 2: Intervention with the Child
1. Help child feel that soiling is a problem that can be solved
2. Help relieve guilt feelings if present

Step 3: Intervention with the Parents
1. Help parents ventilate frustration, anger, or guilt
2. Help parents understand that soiling is not usually intentional
3. Explain that punitive approaches will not help the problem
4. Teach toilet training methods, if needed
5. Assess whether conflict within the family may be contributing to the problem (consider Step 5, below).

Step 4: Use of reinforcers
1. Give a special privilege (e.g., allow child to play with a favorite toy) for defecating in appropriate place
2. Give child some responsibility for cleaning self when soiling occurs

Step 5: Refer to mental health specialist if:
- No improvement after six weeks
- Encopresis is found to be voluntary (e.g., if child seems to soil to provoke parents) and/or major family conflict is present.

Figure 18.4. Encopresis, management

chance to ventilate frustration, anger or guilt, and helping them to understand that punitive approaches toward the child will not alleviate the problem. Parents may need encouragement to express their feelings about the problem. Normally the child's soiling is not intentional and parental understanding of this will reduce parents' feelings or belief that the child should be punished. When soiling is intentional and is being used by the child to provoke parents (e.g., smearing feces on a wall, or soiling just after a parental reminder to go to the bathroom), referral to a mental health specialist for therapy, preferably family therapy, is indicated. In therapy, the psychological needs of the child should be investigated and alternate ways of gratifying such needs identified. For some, increased contact between the father and child may be important.

When soiling seems to have been associated with very little toilet training, providing basic instruction in toilet training is the obvious form of intervention. Instruction can be given on how the bowel works and an understanding communicated that weak muscles can be strengthened. For situations in which toilet training has been overly harsh, the approach to the parents involves teaching them to train the child in a more relaxed way. The child may have to be desensitized to fears of the toilet experience. For a young child, having a small potty-chair to carry around with him may be helpful; for the older child, taking a favorite toy, puzzle, or book to the bathroom, playing special music or talking with the child could help him feel more comfortable. Such efforts require repetition on a daily basis.

For the child with other handicaps, such as hyperactivity or mental retardation (depending on the severity), the use of reinforcers, such as a special privilege, for defecation in the appropriate place can be helpful. Behavior modification is helpful with most of the encopretic children. It is important to have the child identify the reinforcers (experiences or items) that are valuable to him or her. Also, having the child assume responsibility for cleaning up himself or herself (while the parents continue to take care of the laundry) can help the child assume some responsibility for the soiling behavior. Communication of sympathy toward the parents for their plight can help alleviate their burden.

STUTTERING

Stuttering is a disorder characterized by interruption in the flow of speech. Repetition of initial vowels or consonants in syllables or words may be the problem, or, due to muscle spasms, there may be intermittent difficulty with articulating sounds at all. Stuttering is found in 1% of the population, more frequently in boys than girls, and it tends to persist longer in boys. There seems to be a familial tendency towards stuttering and it is also associated with slower acquisition of motor skills. The cause of stuttering is not known, but it is believed to be associated with emotional stress.

Clinical Picture

The onset of stuttering tends to be between eight months and 9 years of age, with peaks of onset between the ages of 2 to 3½ and 5 to 7 years. Many preschool children evidence speech problems in the process of acquiring language skills, which tend to disappear if there is little focus on them. About 50% to 80% of children who stutter outgrow it without special intervention. Around age 3, about 10% of children stutter, but for half of these children the problem will disappear spontaneously. In the older child, stuttering may be precipitated by a frightening event such as an operation or an accident. Stuttering may be constantly an issue or may occur in selected situations, such as being called on in school.

Stuttering may be due to anxiety in the child, associated with parents who

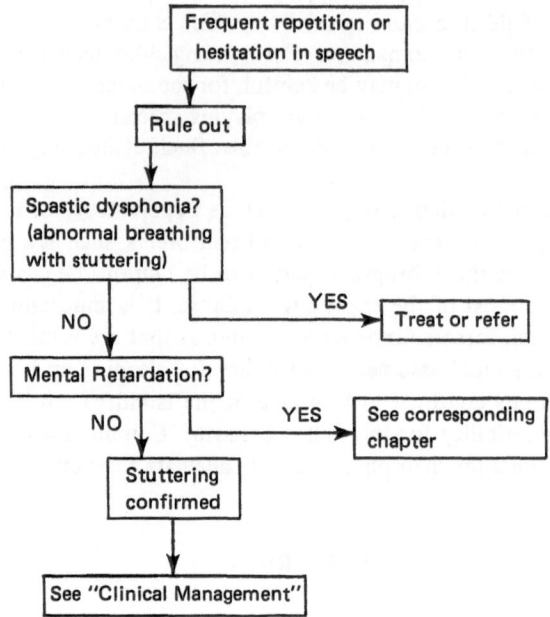

Figure 18.5. Stuttering, diagnostic flow chart

Intervention with Parents

1. Encourage parents to pay attention to *what* the child says rather than how he or she speaks;
2. Tell parents not to prompt the child or to speak for him or her;
3. Emphasize the need for patience to avoid raising the child's level of anxiety.

Referral

1. Refer the child to a speech therapist to unlearn problematic speech patterns if no progress in three months.
2. Refer to a mental health specialist only if secondary problems, such as extreme shyness, develop.

Figure 18.6. Stuttering, management

are perfectionistic and demanding. As attention is drawn to the hesitant or repetitive speech, parental efforts to help the child speak correctly frequently result in reinforcing the stuttering, thereby increasing the problem. The harder the child tries to please his parents, the worse the speech becomes. As the child begins to recognize that he or she is different from others, secondary effects such as avoiding people may develop.

Diagnosis

The diagnosis of stuttering normally requires a brief conversation with the child, although obtaining a parental report of special circumstances or sounds that the child has difficulty with is also necessary. Diagnostic criteria include: "frequent repetitions or prolongation of sounds, syllables, or words or frequent, unusual hesitations and pauses that disrupt the rhythmic flow of speech" (DSM-III, p. 79). The differential diagnosis for stuttering is simple. The diagnosis of a speech problem should not be made if it is a symptom of severe mental retardation. Also, spastic dysphonia is distinguished from stuttering by an abnormal pattern of breathing.

Clinical Management

The major focus of the health professional's work with the child's parents is to provide education and reassurance. If parents can be taught to concentrate on what the child is saying rather than how the child is speaking, speech in the young child will most likely improve with the child's growth. Parents have to learn to resist their urge to help the child either by prompting or speaking for the child. Instead, patience on the parents' part which gives sufficient time for the child to get out what he is trying to say, can prevent the anxiety associated with speaking. The health professional can contribute significantly by encouraging a sense of optimism in the parents.

If stuttering gets worse or does not improve after a reasonable period of time, referral to a speech therapist to help the child unlearn problematic speech patterns is advised. Referral to a mental health specialist is usually not needed unless secondary effects of stuttering, such as extreme shyness or low self-esteem, require therapeutic intervention. There are cases of stuttering that are very refractory to change, even after intensive treatment. In such cases, hypnosis has been reported helpful as an adjunct therapeutic modality.

CHAPTER 19

Mental Retardation

Mental retardation is characterized by significantly below average intellectual functioning (intelligence below 70), with deficits in social and emotional functioning and onset before the age of 18. Causal factors may be biological, sociopsychological, or both. The prevalence of mental retardation in the general population is estimated at 1%. Higher rates are reported among school-age children, who are recognized through standardized testing of academic achievement and intellectual functioning. Mental retardation is twice as common among males as among females. The great majority (87%) of retarded individuals fall into the mildly retarded group (IQ 51-70) and come predominantly from the lower socioeconomic classes. Their retardation is believed to be a function of environmental deprivation. Among the more severe forms of retardation, the lower socioeconomic groups are more highly represented, but not as disproportionately as among the milder forms.

CLINICAL PICTURE

From social and psychological perspectives, mental retardation is seen as developmental impairment in infancy, as learning difficulties in the school-age child, and as poor social and vocational adjustment in adolescence and adulthood. Mildly retarded children can be educated to a limited extent (usually to a sixth-grade level) and are potentially able to adjust at least minimally to the demands of society. The moderately mentally retarded (IQ 35-49) can learn to talk and communicate and can profit from training in social and occupational skills, but are unlikely to achieve beyond a second-grade level in academic subjects. The severely retarded (IQ 20-34) are not likely to develop speech until school-age and as adults may only be expected to perform simple repetitive tasks under close supervision. The profoundly mentally retarded, who constitute only 1% of retarded individuals, require a highly structured environment with constant aid and supervision, although limited motor and speech development may occur from the school-age period through adulthood.

The course of mental retardation is closely tied to whether a specific biological abnormality is present. The milder forms, due to psychosocial deprivation, may be responsive to remedial approaches, while retardation associated with a biological insult is usually chronic and without remission. Biological bases of mental retardation are multiple and may occur at prenatal, perinatal, or postnatal periods. Retardation with a prenatal basis tends to have its origin in metabolic and chromosomal disorders. One of each group, phenylketonuria (PKU), and Down's syndrome, are described below. (For information on related disorders see Cytryn and Lourie, 1980.)

PKU

When untreated, PKU (phenylketonuria) presents with severe retardation, an abnormal electroencephalogram and seizures, hyperactivity, and poor coordination and communication. Physical signs include a light complexion, small head, and coarse features. If treated within 3 to 6 months of birth with a low-phenylalanine diet, the potential of normal or near-normal intelligence can be realized; also, the child will be more responsive and less hyperactive than if untreated. The dietary treatment is not always without complications, which may include anemia, hypoglycemia, or edema.

Down's syndrome

Among the chromosomal disorders, Down's syndrome has been extensively researched. This disorder is the result of trisomy of the 21st chromosome. The incidence of births with Down's syndrome is 1 in 700. In mothers over 32 years of age there is a risk of 1 in 100, but when translocation (fusion of two chromosomes, usually 15 and 21) is present, the risk of Down's syndrome is 1 in 3—an implication for genetic counseling. The clinical picture is generally one of moderate to severe retardation, although children with few symptoms may develop normal or superior ability. Some 100 symptoms are seen in Down's syndrome, but not all of them are found in any single child. Notable symptoms include slanting eyes, a protruding tongue, broad, thick hands, and the absence of the Moro reflex. No treatment has proven effective. These children tend to be placid, cheerful, and cooperative during childhood, and their life expectancy has increased significantly due to the availability of antibiotics.

Complications during pregnancy may also contribute to mental retardation. Maternal diabetes presents hazards, as does the use of certain pharmacological agents and substance abuse (e.g., fetal alcohol syndrome). In the perinatal period, premature birth with low birthweight (below 3 lbs. 4 ounces) usually results in intellectual deficits, sensory and motor handicaps, convulsive disorders and learning and emotional difficulties. Other cerebral insults may occur with breech delivery, abnormal presentation requiring use of midforceps and high forceps, prolonged labor, and anoxia associated with cesarean section or respiratory difficulty caused by analgesic and anesthetic drugs.

In the postnatal period, a number of other biological factors can cause retardation. These include meningitis (if unrecognized and untreated); lead poisoning resulting from pica; trauma such as head injuries. (The latter seldom produce retardation, however.) Other disorders such as epilepsy (20-25% of the retarded living in institutions) and cerebral palsy (less than 15% of cerebral palsy patients have normal intelligence) are associated with retardation.

Malnutrition, involving early caloric and protein deficiencies, affects growth and will produce irreversible changes in mental functioning, including retardation. Some degree of retardation associated with sociocultural conditions in backward rural communities and urban slums may occur in 10-30% of the population. Contributing factors include little or no prenatal care, poor nutrition, and infections during pregnancy, a higher rate of premature births, understimulation or overstimulation of the child, and poor nutrition of the child, complicated by social problems such as disturbed family relationships and inconsistent limit-setting.

DIAGNOSIS

The diagnostic process starts with the primary health care practitioner, but also frequently requires the involvement of other specialists. The primary care provider should investigate the following:

1. History of pregnancy, labor, delivery, and hereditary disorders in the family.
2. Developmental milestones (see Chapter 13). Recognize that parents may distort due to bias and anxiety.
3. The emotional climate of the family and sociocultural background.
4. Physical signs, such as the size of the child's head, facial size, and the overall size of the child.
5. Adequacy of vision, hearing, and speech.
6. Neurological signs, including muscle tone, involuntary movement, sensory disturbance, hyperactivity, short attention span, distractibility, and frustration tolerance.

Further evaluations might require an ophthalmologist, audiologist, speech and language specialist, and a neurologist. Evaluation by a psychiatrist can be useful to assess the stage of personality development, and an experienced psychologist is required to assess intellectual functioning. The most widely accepted intelligence tests used by psychologists are the Stanford-Binet and the Wechsler Intelligence Scale for Children (WISC). The Peabody Vocabulary Test is an acceptable alternative for children without communications or tactile skills.

The following diagnostic questionnaire relies upon the results of the preceding assessments, including the psychological evaluation.

QUESTIONNAIRE FOR MENTAL RETARDATION

	YES	NO
1. Is the child's level of intellectual functioning below an IQ of 70 or, in the case of infants, judged as subaverage functioning ? (In most cases testing by a psychologist is required to answer this question.)	——	—
2. Is the child's social and emotional functioning (e.g., relationships with peers and siblings, patterns of play) well below what would be expected for his/her age level? This can usually be assessed by the health professional, based on his/her knowledge of developmental tasks.	——	—

If the answers to the preceding questions are YES, it is necessary to rule out the following conditions, which would normally be detected through the above-suggested evaluations: (1) A physical handicap, such as blindness, deafness, cerebral palsy, or speech problems, which may make the child seem retarded; (2) chronic disease, such as convulsive disorders, which may depress intellectual functioning; (3) chronic brain syndrome, which may produce an isolated handicap as opposed to overall retardation; (4) emotional difficulty, which may cause the child to do poorly and present with apparent retardation; (5) other mental disorder—in infantile autism or childhood schizophrenia the child may appear retarded, however, the differential diagnosis is not significant initially; the first treatment step in either case is to help the child learn to relate to others.

CLINICAL MANAGEMENT

Following diagnosis, which in most cases will require the assistance of other professionals, intervention by the health professional with the parents is critical, whatever the cause of retardation. Producing a handicapped child frequently contributes to feelings of inadequacy on the part of the parents, including grief over the loss of the normal child that was expected. The child's lack of responsiveness to parental efforts leads to feelings of disappointment in the parents and may result in either a parental response of rejection or overprotection of the child. Following diagnosis of a child, anguish and tension at home make this a

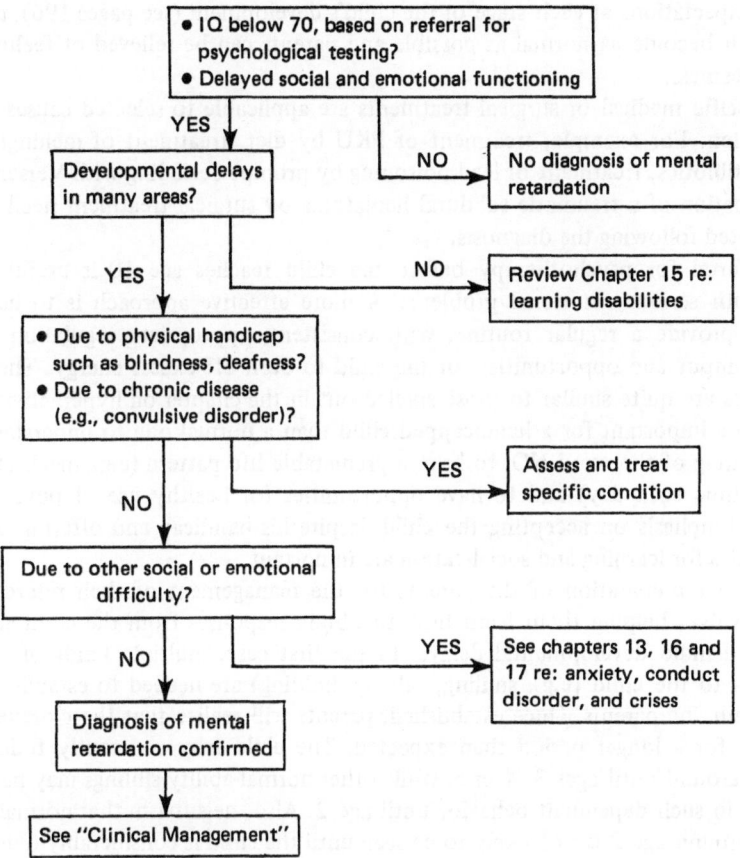

Figure 19.1. Mental retardation, diagnostic flow chart

particularly crucial time for the family. Further, the limited social life of the family associated with the care of the retarded child or fearfulness of rejection by others frequently results in social isolation of the whole family.

The health provider can play an important role in preventing tension within the family through providing clarification of the expected extent of handicap, support around increased duties of the parents, and reassurance, as appropriate, regarding the child's future. The health professional needs to be realistic about limitations in relation to a given level of ability, but can help parents understand that most retarded children can live both a satisfying and useful life. The health professional's communication of concern and interest can help bring out the parents' feelings and attitudes. Through guidance that offers specific information about expectations at each stage of the child's development (see pages 196), the child can become as normal as possible and parents can be relieved of feelings of helplessness.

Specific medical or surgical treatments are applicable to selected causes of retardation. For example, treatment of PKU by diet, treatment of meningitis with antibiotics, treatment of lead poisoning by prompt deleading with Versene, or evacuation of a traumatic subdural hematoma by surgical treatment need to be initiated following the diagnosis.

Referral for psychotherapy before the child reaches age 10 is useful in cases with serious emotional problems. A more effective approach is to help parents provide a regular routine, with consistent, appropriate regulation of sensory input and opportunities for the child to burn off excess energy. These principles are quite similar to those spelled out in the chapter on hyperactivity. It is more important for a handicapped child than a normal one to understand the meaning of the word NO, to have a predictable life pattern (e.g., meals at a regular time each day) and to have opportunities for healthy use of physical energy. Emphasis on accepting the child despite his handicap and offering opportunities for learning and socialization are important.

Further preparation of the parents for the management of their retarded child involves helping them learn how to obtain responses from the child and how to handle developmental delays. In the first case, multiple kinds of approaches to the child (e.g., smiling, talking, holding) are needed to establish a bond with the parents. Once established, parents will realize that the closeness goes on for a longer period than expected. The child may constantly follow mother around until ages 3, 4 or 5, while other normal-ability siblings may have engaged in such dependent behavior until age 2. Also, negativism that normally occurs around age 2 is not likely to be seen until the child is considerably older, necessitating that parents avoid head-on confrontations with an older child. While constant "NO's" from a two-year old might be acceptable to parents, such behavior in an older child requires reminders to parents that this is normal for a retarded child.

As the child gets older and displays problems either with his or her self-image or with behavior, further therapeutic considerations may be in order. Group therapy for the child can facilitate communication of feelings, help the child obtain acceptance from peers, and reinforce acceptable behavior. Behavior modification approaches have been developed to change specific behavior through a process of identifying problematic behaviors, breaking the behavior into small parts, and developing rewards that recognize behavioral change. For the parents, continued guidance by the health provider through the difficult phase of raising the child is necessary. Channeling parental frustration into a group of parents who have retarded children or helping to plan periodic relief from child care through day care, summer camp, or temporary institutionalization are part of the ongoing counseling role of the health professional.

Table 19.1   Clinical Management Instructions for Mental Retardation

1. Following the diagnosis of mental retardation, working closely with parents around the following initial tasks is crucial:

    a. Helping parents acknowledge feelings about having a handicapped child.
    b. Teach parents how to relate to the child to obtain a response from the child.
    c. Encourage the family to continue normal social activities and reassure them that time away from the child is important.
    d. Provide information on expected delays in the child's social development and management approaches that will help the child develop as normally as possible.

2. For retardation in which there is effective medical treatment, such as diet in the case of PKU, ensure that parents understand the potential benefits of the dietary regimen and monitor the child closely.
3. If the older retarded child exhibits a poor self-image (e.g., makes derogatory comments about self), or behavioral problems, consider a referral for group therapy or behavior modification.
4. As the child gets older, continue to assess parental acceptance and management of the child and help parents find support through a group for parents of retarded children.
5. By preschool or minimally at school age, the health professional can work with school personnel to obtain needed special-education services.
6. In the case of the profoundly retarded child who cannot be managed adequately at home, institutional placement may have to be considered.
7. Emphasize the child's strengths and help parents recognize gains throughout the child's growth and development.
8. Long-term planning for vocational training should begin by early adolescence with a focus on decreasing the patient's dependence on the family. Placement in sheltered workshops and a group home may provide additional alternatives during early adult years.

Finally, providing information and intervening with school officials to obtain special services such as a special educational placement for the child is a legitimate role for the health professional. This involves helping parents find a preschool and later a school-age program that will build on the child's assets: take into account the need for repetition and any sensory handicaps; stress prevocational experiences; and include behavior modification approaches, depending upon the specific needs of the child. A long-range plan aimed at developing the greatest independence possible in social and occupational functioning requires regular meetings over time between the health professional, parents and child. While continuing to be realistic with parents about the child or young adult's potential, it is important to identify school and work experiences that will promote pride and accomplishment to the extent possible. For example, in a very low-ability individual, this could mean placement in a sheltered workshop with intensive supervision, while for young adults who are moderately handicapped, a job requiring less supervision should be encouraged. Particularly since the overall process is characterized by ups and downs for the child and the family, a continuous emphasis on the strengths of the child and his or her gains is most important.

REFERENCES

Cytryn L, Lourie RS. Mental Retardation. In: *Comprehensive Textbook of Psychiatry*, Vol. 3, 3rd Edition. Kaplan HI, Freedman AM, Sadock BJ (Eds.). Baltimore: Williams & Wilkins, 1980.

Kock R, Dobson JC (Eds.). *The Mentally Retarded Child and His Family*. New York: Brunner/Mazel, 1980.

Menolascino FJ (Ed.). *Psychiatric Aspects of the Diagnosis and Treatment of Mental Retardation*. New York: Basic Books, 1970.

Psychopharmacology

PSYCHOPHARMACOLOGY

Most of the psychopharmacological products discussed in this chapter are intended for adults and older adolescents; for children, as appropriate, the discussion is included in each chapter. The present chapter includes antidepressants, antipsychotics, minor tranquilizers and antiparkinsonians. The anticonvulsants are discussed in Chapter 8. A combined discussion of the different psychopharmacological products used in daily practice is intended to provide greater flexibility for comparison of different drugs and different alternatives. It is not infrequent, for example, that some of the drugs described in the text are either not available or not tolerated by some patients, requiring the clinician to be knowledgeable about a limited number of equivalent products. This chapter should serve as a guide in such cases; the management of the most common situations should stem from material presented in the preceding chapters. The generic name of a drug is used due to the multiplicity of commercial drug names. If necessary, the reader is referred to the commercial list (see Table 20.1).

The psychopharmacological emphasis in this chapter and in the specific psychopharmacological discussions in each chapter, is focused on drugs with known efficacy for the relief of severe and incapacitating symptoms. In each chapter the social and psychological components of each disorder that can be handled effectively at the primary health care level have been described. Comprehensive and biopsychosocial management of each problem should be always kept in mind. This should not rule out the possibility that in some cases treatment may be primarily biological, psychological or social; in the vast majority of cases, however, a multiple approach towards alleviating the problem is more desirable.

Table 20.1 Most Common Commercial Names of Psychopharmacological
Products

Generic Name	Commercial Name (and Manufacturer)
ANTIDEPRESSANTS	
Amitriptyline	Elavil (Merck, Sharp & Dohme)
Desipramine HCl	Pertofrane (USV Pharmaceutical)
	Norpramin (Merrell Dow)
Imipramine HCl	Tofranil (Geigy)
ANTIPSYCHOTICS	
High-Dosage	
Chlorpromazine	Thorazine (Smith, Kline & French)
Thioridazine HCl	Mellaril (Sandoz)
Low-Dosage	
Haloperidol	Haldol (McNeil)
Trifluoperazine	Stelazine (Smith, Kline & French)
Fluphenazine	Permitil (Schering)
	Prolixin (Squibb)
ANXIOLYTICS (MINOR TRANQUILIZERS)	
Diazepam	Valium (Roche)
Chlordiazepoxide	Librium (Roche)
ANTIPARKINSONIANS	
Biperiden	Akineton (Knoll)
Trihexyphenidyl	Artane (Lederle)
	Tremin (Schering)

A frequently underestimated factor of failure in the use of these medications is noncompliance; this should be carefully reviewed in each case. Noncompliance can take one of several forms: the patient refuses to take the prescribed dosage; the patient initiates the treatment but, after initial improvement, abandons the treatment; the patient uses secondary side effects as an excuse to discontinue medication; at the end of the first prescription the patient loses interest in the treatment. Noncompliance is not likely to change without the physician's inquiring directly about the exact number of tablets taken. He may count the number of tablets still left in the bottle and investigate the schedule used for taking the medication. If such procedures are not carried out properly, the patient is not likely to improve and the clinician will be unable to determine the cause of treatment failure.

Other factors enhancing the possibility of the success of psychopharmacological agents involve the proper selection of the drug, adequate dosage for the specific clinical problem, a sufficiently long trial period, and adequate follow-up, as well as attention to secondary and toxic effects.

ANTIDEPRESSANTS

One group of antidepressants, the tricyclics, including the three families most frequently prescribed, will be discussed: amitriptyline, desipramine, and imipramine. Other antidepressants, such as the monoaminoxide inhibitors (MAOI), will not be discussed, due to the relative complexities in management (e.g., diet restrictions, incompatibility with other drugs). Trazodone, a new, promising antidepressant, is mentioned as an interesting drug with few side effects and reduced cardiotoxicity.

Amitriptyline

Depression with anxiety and insomnia (without psychomotor retardation) is the most frequent type of depression in clinical practice. The drug of choice is amitriptyline, 25 mg tablets P.O., before bedtime; its antianxiety properties help the patient to relax, inducing sleep.

Initially, one tablet for one or two days at bedtime should provide an indication of individual tolerance. If the drug is well tolerated and there are no bothersome side effects, the dosage is increased to 50 mg for two days, followed by gradual increments up to 100 mg/day. In cases in which moderate improvement and a good tolerance are observed, an increase of up to 150 mg per day may be considered. The entire daily dosage may be given at bedtime or may be divided in two periods of about 8–12 hours each.

Desipramine

For depression with psychomotor retardation, fatigue, or disinterest, but without a marked component of anxiety or insomnia, the antidepressant of choice of desipramine, 25 mg tablets, P.O., in the mornings. It is not recommended after midday, since it can produce insomnia.

Initiate with one 25-mg tablet during 1 to 2 days, to test tolerance and side effects. If the patient is not bothered by severe side effects, two tablets for two additional days are followed by 3 tablets per day thereafter. If there is clinical improvement after the first week without side effects, the dosages may be increased to up to 100 mg/day or even up to 150 mg/day. The average patient improves considerably with a dosage of about 75 mg to 150 mg per day.

IMIPRAMINE

Trial period and follow-up

The tricyclic antidepressants require adequate trial periods. Three weeks are required before the antidepressant's effects are fully evident. Discontinuation before this period is therefore not recommended, unless severe side effects develop. This should be presented to the patient convincingly in order to prevent early withdrawal.

Change of antidepressants

It is possible that during the trial period the patient will show bothersome side effects that force the clinician to discontinue medication; in these cases the physician should be advised to change to another compound. For example, if the patient suffers a depression associated with anxiety and has not tolerated amitriptyline, imipramine may be tried. Imipramine may also be used in depression with psychomotor retardation if desipramine is not tolerated by the patient. If the patient does not show improvement after three weeks of treatment, a referral to a specialist is in order. Follow-up of these medications after clinical improvement should be maintained at least for three months; drug withdrawal after a complete stabilization of the clinical symptoms should be gradual.

Secondary and toxic effects

The tricyclic antidepressants are drugs to be handled with great caution for several reasons:

(1) therapeutic dosages pose a greater risk than for most of the commonly used psychopharmacological agents;

(2) these drugs are used in persons with a higher suicidal potential than the average patient;

(3) during the recovery phase, the patient may mobilize latent suicidal thoughts as well as the strength to carry out suicidal acts; this is one of the reasons why close observation of the suicidal patient must be continued beyond the initial clinical improvement;

(4) the suicidal danger is high in these patients; therefore, the prescription of over 20 tablets (500 mg) at a time is not recommended. Forty tablets (or 10000 mg) has been considered a lethal dosage;

(5) the lack of control in the sale of antidepressants in some places poses further problems;

The above reasons indicate the need for precautions in the use of antidepressants especially among debilitated and older individuals; they are contraindicated in heart, liver, CNS (i.e., epilepsy) disorders and narrow-angle glaucoma.

Secondary effects include sedation and dizziness, which can be quite limiting and bothersome and especially pronounced at the beginning of treatment. Other common side effects include dryness of mouth, constipation, perspiration, and blurred vision; also, cardiac arrhythmias, orthostatic hypotension or hypertension (less common). Urinary retention, insomnia, fine hand tremors, and weight increase. The latter effects can be of brief duration and most of them improve with time; they should not necessarily result in withdrawal of the drug, unless severity is marked. Other, much less frequent but more severe side effects include those of the CNS (i.e., tremors, agitation, delusions, and/or hallucinations). Overdoses of these drugs could be treated with physostigmine 1–4 mg I.M. or I.V.

ANTIPSYCHOTICS

The high- and low-dosage antipsychotic agents will be discussed. The prototype of high-dosage antipsychotics is chlorpromazine. The low-dosage drugs include, among others, haloperidol and trifluoperazine.

Chlorpromazine

This phenothiazine is the most widely used antipsychotic, despite the fact that in the U.S. it seems to be replaced by other drugs (i.e., haloperidol). It is an excellent drug when the psychotic patient requires sedation (i.e., for the agitated psychotic). Its disadvantages include tardive dyskinesia, cardiovascular effects, orthostatic hypotension, and tachycardia, as well as various extrapyramidal effects and muscle dystonias.

Haloperidol

Haloperidol is a butyrophenone that appears to be replacing chlorpromazine in the psychopharmacological management of acute psychosis. While it is less sedating than chlorpromazine, the antipsychotic effects are comparable.

Trifluoperazine

This low-dosage phenothiazine is useful in the management of psychotic patients without much agitation, and its use appears to be more effective when there are thought disturbances, hallucinations, delusions, and paranoid ideations.

The low-dosage antipsychotic agents produce less hypotension and less sedation, but extrapyramidal effects are more pronounced than with the high-dosage products. Trifluoperazine, if used at high dosages, almost invariably requires the simultaneous use of antiparkinsonian medications.

Indications for Use of Antipsychotics

Patients with a better chance of a positive response to antipsychotics include: those with acute rather than chronic psychotic episodes; those with a great increase in motor activity, insomnia, poor appetite, hallucinations and delusions. Antipsychotics are also useful in less severe psychosis during relapses of previous psychotic episodes. Chances of improvement are understandably greater when patients comply with recommended drug regimens. The most common clinical pictures found in psychosis are:

Acute psychosis

Frequently, an acutely psychotic patient shows psychomotor agitation; ideas of control, reference, persecution, grandeur; hallucinations; delusions; thought disorders; neologisms, hostility and/or insomnia.

If the patient does not cooperate, an alternative could be haloperidol 5 mg I.M. Repeat every hour to a maximum of 40 mg, or until symptoms are controlled or sedation is adequate. If patient is cooperative, use haloperidol tablets 10 mg P.O., up to 40 mg per day in two dosages; be careful of side effects and oversedation.

One alternative drug that could be used if the patient does not cooperate is chlorpromazine 25 mg, one or two ampules I.M. in one administration. This dose may be repeated every half-hour up to a maximum of 200 mg, or until agitation improves. If the patient is cooperative the same psychotherapeutic principles as in Chapter 11 ("Psychosis") are kept in mind and the following psychopharmacological program is used: chlorpromazine 25-mg tablets, 3 per day at bedtime on the first day; progressive increase up to 400 mg per day. If there is no improvement, refer to a mental health specialist.

Subacute psychosis

The patient shows psychotic symptomatology with ideas of control, reference, persecution and/or grandeur and/or hallucinations and/or delusional ideas, and/or thought disorders, and/or neologisms, and/or insomnia, *but* agitation is not marked and the patient appears willing to cooperate with treatment.

Chlorpromazine 25-mg tablets, as used in acute psychosis, is one possibility. In a cooperative patient, dosages of up to 100-300 mg/day should be the upper limit. Another possibility is trifluoperazine 5-mg tablets, 3 tablets per day. Due to its notorious extrapyramidal effects, antiparkinsonian drugs are almost invariably required with chlorpromazine (see Chapter 11, "Psychosis").

Chronic psychosis

Most of the symptoms of acute psychosis are found in the chronic forms, but there is no agitation and the symptoms have developed over a longer period. Patients may have been suffering from these symptoms for months or even years with chronic social difficulties, and they may even have a history of repeated psychiatric hospitalizations. In chronic psychosis, the drug of choice is fluphenazine 2-5 mg, 2 times per day tablets P.O. Increases should be gradual in order to determine tolerance; once the therapeutic level is established, the dosage could be maintained at approximately 4 mg, twice a day for several months. If the patient is uncooperative, long-acting products are indicated such as fluphenazine enanthate or fluphenazine decanoate; they should be prescribed by a psychiatrist.

An alternative to the above is trifluoperazine 5 mg tablets, 15 mg per day. Because of the need for long treatment through several-times-a-day administration, trifluoperazine will more frequently result in noncompliance than will the long-acting products.

Lithium carbonate is the drug of choice in the manic phase of the manic depressive disorder. It is not discussed in this volume due to the complications of its use and the need for blood-level monitoring, which is generally difficult at the primary health care level. Manic-depressive patients should be referred to a mental health specialist.

Testing Period for Antipsychotic Drugs

The testing period for the antipsychotic drugs should be 1-2 weeks. Most of the antipsychotic drugs have an immediate sedative action; nevertheless, their effect on hallucinations or delusions begins to be noticeable several days or even weeks after the initiation of treatment. Relatives should be advised of this fact. Side effects are more frequent at the beginning of treatment, i.e., hypotension, arrhythmias, extrapyramidal effects, oversedation, and muscle dystonias. Advise patient and relatives regarding the fact that these problems will probably disappear with time, since such information may prevent a premature withdrawal from treatment.

Resistance to Treatment with Antipsychotics

Many times, when no relief from psychotic symptoms is obtained through the use of a medication, there is a tendency to blame failure on the specific drug and to seek a different one. Be reminded that the most common cause of treatment failure is noncompliance. It is important to establish objectively the real drug intake, in order to gather adequate information regarding treatment. The next step is to increase the dosage and to wait a few days; if the initial dosage is high, it could be reduced as a last step before making the decision to switch to another drug, because it is possible that toxicity may be interfering with the therapeutic effects; if there is no improvement, a change is justified.

Table 20.2 Recommended Dosages and Indications of the Most Frequently Used Psychopharmacological Products.

	P.O. Utilization (mg in 24 hours) Initial	Maintenance	Indications	I.M. Utilization (mg/24 hrs)	Indications
ANTIDEPRESSANTS					
Amitriptyline	25	75-150	Depression with anxiety + insomnia; without retardation.	—	—
Desipramine	25	75-100	Depression with retardation without major anxiety.	—	—
Imipramine	25	75-150	Depression without major anxiety or retardation.	—	—
ANTIPSYCHOTICS High-Dosage:					
Chlorpromazine	75	300-400	Acute psychosis with agitation.	50-200	*Marked agitation* I.M. use every half-hour X 3.

Low-Dosage:					
Haloperidol	5-10	10-40	Acute psychosis with moderate agitation.	5-40	Same as above
Trifluoperazine	5	15	Chronic psychosis with paranoid delusions.	—	—
Fluphenazine	2-4	4-8	Same as above.	—	—
ANXIOLYTICS					
Diazepam	5	5-15	Anxiety (without psychosis or depression).	5-20	Alcohol withdrawal. Status epilepticus.
Chlordiazepoxide	10-50	15-200	Same as above.	—	Same as above.
ANTIPARKINSONIANS					
Biperiden	2	2-8	Parkinsonian symptoms, muscle dystonias.	2-8	Acute dystonias, Marked akathisia
Trihexyphenidyl	2	2-10	Same as above.	—	Same as above.

Time of administration: antidepressants, antipsychotics and anxiolytics are administered at bedtime in single dosages; maximum in two daily administrations.
Exception: Desipramine should be taken in the morning.
Antiparkinsonians: in two daily dosages.

Secondary Effects of Antipsychotic Drugs

Cardiovascular effects

Orthostatic hypotension is common with antipsychotics. The typical symptom is sudden dizziness when the patient gets up; this may be prevented by suggesting that the patient stand up slowly, and it improves when the patient sits or lies down. Tachycardia is also mentioned as a side effect of antipsychotics.

Central nervous system effects

Any antipsychotic could trigger grand mal seizures; therefore, they should be used with caution in persons with a history of epilepsy. The most common side effect of the phenothiazine group is pseudoparkinsonism, a syndrome that includes a stiff robotlike gait, lack of spontaneity, a fixed facial expression, and motor restlessness.

Autonomic nervous system effects

Dryness of the mouth, blurred vision, difficulties in urination, and in severe cases, urinary retention are among the autonomic nervous system effects of antipsychotic drugs.

Other side effects

Muscle dystonias generally associated with pseudoparkinsonism are characterized by muscle contractions, stiffness or twisting of body parts; also akathisia, characterized by intense restlessness (the patient walks and moves incessantly). Dermatitis due to sun exposure is common with the use of chlorpromazine; weight increase occurs when treatment is carried out for relatively long periods; retarded ejaculation and galactorrhea are also associated with the use of chlorpromazine.

Tardive dyskinesia is a progressive, generally irreversible syndrome that appears as a reaction to the use of antipsychotics. It is characterized by movements of the lips, protrusion of the tongue, as well as abnormal movements of other facial muscles. The movements are perioral, as if the patient were rinsing the mouth or chewing. Frequent movement of the eyes and exaggerated gestures also occur. The most effective procedure to handle this problem is prevention; treatment with antipsychotics should include the minimum effective dosage for the minimum length of time (a difficult decision, since there is no clear agreement as to adequate maintenance periods). Decreasing or discontinuing the medication when the first signs of dyskinesia appear may help, although in many situations the initial appearance of the symptoms already constitute an irreversible situation. Antiparkinsonians are not recommended since they tend to worsen the problem.

Table-20.3   Side Effects of the Most Commonly Used Psychopharmacological Products

Side Effects	Anti-depres-sants	Antipsychotics High-Dose	Low-Dose	Anxio-lytics	Anti-parkin-sonians
Autonomic Effects					
Blurred vision	*	**	*	o	*
Dry mouth	**	***	*	o	o
Constipation	**	*	*	o	*
Urinary retention	**	*	*	o	*
Sweatness	*	*	*	o	o
Cardiovascular Effects					
Orthostatic hypotension	*	***	*	o	o
Tachycardia	*	*	*	o	o
Hypertension	o	*	*	o	o
Arrhythmias	o	o	o	o	o
CNS					
Parkinsonism	o	*	***	o	o
Muscle dystonias	o	*	***	o	o
Akathisia	o	*	***	o	o
Convulsions (rare)	*	*	*	o	o
Fine hand tremors	*	o	o	o	o
Other					
Hepatotoxic	*	*	o	o	o
Dermatitis (+)	o	**	o	o	o
Pigmentary retinitis (++)	o	***	o	o	o
Addiction	o	o	o	***	*
Menstrual irregularities	o	**	o	o	o
Galactorrhea	o	**	o	o	o
Increased weight	*	**	o	o	o
Agranulocitosis	*	*	*	o	o
Aggravated glaucoma	***	o	o	o	o
-Suicidal potential	***	o	o	**	o
-Tardive dyskinesia (++)	o	***	***	o	o
-Greater intolerance in older or debilitated persons	**	**	*	**	o
-Toxic psychosis	*	*	o	**	*
-Insomnia	*	o	o	o	o
-Dizziness	*	*	*	o	o
-Oversedation	*	*	*	o	o
-Extrapyramidal effects	o	*	*	o	o

Chlorpromazine (+)
Thioridazine   (++)
Chronic use   (+++)
Code: o = usually absent; * = minimum; ** = moderate; *** = marked.

Toxic effects

The antipsychotics have a low toxicity if properly used. A phenothiazine particularly useful in psychotic depression is thioridazine, but it is not discussed in detail in this chapter due to the remote possibility of causing pigmentary retinitis. Toxic effects of other drugs are rare but can include CNS depression with temperature control loss; marked hypotension, especially in debilitated or elderly patients.

ANXIOLYTICS (MINOR TRANQUILIZERS)

Minor tranquilizers are widely used for the management of acute or chronic forms of anxiety. They may also be used in the management of acute insomnia, in alcohol withdrawal syndrome, or in status epilepticus. These drugs are *not* utilized in psychosis or depression because they are not effective, since their use can result in addiction; if a prescription is necessary, it should be for a limited time. There is a great variety of tranquilizers, but only two products are recommended here for use at the primary health care level: diazepam and chlordiazepoxide. Meprobamate is not recommended, due to its toxicity.

Anxiety

Both diazepam and chlordiazepoxide are minor tranquilizers with specific antianxiety effects, usually well tolerated with relatively low toxicity. Effects are evident 30 minutes after administration. The recommended dosage is 5 mg P.O., one to three times per day; in severe cases this dosage may be doubled. Administration should not exceed 30 mg/day and should be limited to one week. If anxiety is severe (e.g., a panic attack), and if the patient is uncooperative, a single I.M. administration of 10 mg diazepam is useful. If anxiety persists, patients should be referred to a mental health specialist.

Alcohol Withdrawal

The symptoms of severe alcohol withdrawal include alcoholic hallucinosis, delirium tremens, and convulsions. They are all severe clinical conditions considered as medical emergencies that *should not* be managed at primary health care settings. Nevertheless, some knowledge regarding these syndromes is essential in order to make a proper referral. The treatment, whenever possible, should include diazepam 10-20 mg, 3-4 times per day, P.O., up to a maximum of 100 mg per day until the referral is possible. Higher dosages may be utilized, but only under the circumstances of hospitalization.

If P.O. administration cannot be used, while referral to a hospital is possible, diazepam 10-20 mg I.M. may be used. Alternatively, chlordiazepoxide may be used in larger dosages such as 25 mg every 4 hours to sedation; the form of administration is the same as for diazepam.

ANTIPARKINSONIANS

Antiparkinsonians are useful for those symptoms that closely resemble Parkinson's disease, i.e., those appearing as secondary effects of antipsychotic medications (fine hand tremors, muscle rigidity, lack of facial expression, etc.). They are also effective in muscle dystonias and restlessness.

Biperiden and trihexyphenidyl are two antiparkinsonians with similar uses, effects and dosages. Their use is indicated only when the first symptoms are evident. As has been discussed, they are more likely to be necessary if fluphenazine, trifluoperazine, and haloperidol have been prescribed. The symptoms, usually of slow progress, start a few days after the beginning of antipsychotic drugs; even though they are usually bothersome, they constitute no risk to the patient's life. Biperiden or trihexyphenidyl (2-mg tablets) may be used 2-8 mg/day; that is, one or two tablets one to two times per day. Dosages over 10 mg per day are not recommended. In acute dystonias, I.M. antiparkinsonians are desirable. These occur less frequently, but represent a major cause of alarm to the patient due to the acuteness of the symptoms (i.e., torticollis, tongue protrusion or marked akathisia). In these cases, the treatment of choice is biperiden ampules, 2 mg I.M., 1-2 ampules, 1-2 times per day. Maximum dosage is 8 mg per day. Intramuscular administration should be used only during the acute episodes; maintenance should be followed by oral administration of these compounds.

Maintenance

Reduction in dosage of antiparkinsonians can occur after 3 weeks of treatment, with a complete withdrawal of antiparkinsonians if there is no symptom recurrence.

Secondary effects

Due to their anticholinergic effects, the antiparkinsonians may induce or worsen urinary and gastrointestinal problems, especially urinary hesitation or retention and constipation. A certain degree of abuse of these drugs may occur due to the stimulant effects.

Toxic effects

High dosages in sensitive individuals can induce a toxic psychosis with delusional ideas and/or visual and auditory hallucinations.

Overdoses

Overdoses of antiparkinsonians, as for the antidepressants, may be treated with physostigmine 1 to 4 mg I.M. or I.V.

REFERENCES

Appleton WS, Davis JM. *Practical Clinical Psychopharmacology*, 2nd Ed. Baltimore: Williams and Wilkins, 1980.

Bassuk EL, Schoonover SC. *The Practitioner's Guide to Psychoactive Drugs*. New York: Plenum, 1977.

Bowden CL, Giffen, MB. *Psychopharmacology For the Primary Care Physician*. Baltimore: Williams and Wilkens, 1978.

Hollister LE. *Clinical Pharmacology of the Psychoactive Drugs*. New York: Churchill Livingstone, 1978.

Klein DF, Gittelman R, Quitkin F, Rifkin A. *Diagnosis and Treatment of Psychiatric Disorders: Adults and Children*. Baltimore: Williams and Wilkins, 1980.

Lion JR. *The Art of Medicating Psychiatric Patients*. Baltimore: Williams and Wilkins, 1978.

Reid WH. *Psychiatry for the House Officer*. New York: Brunner/Mazel, 1979.

Werry JS. *Pediatric Psychopharmacology: The Use of Behavior-Modifying Drugs in Children and Adolescents*. New York: Brunner/Mazel, 1978.

White JH. *Pediatric Psychopharmacology: A Practical Guide to Clinical Application*. Baltimore: Williams and Wilkins, 1978.

Index

Questionnaire
  for agitation diagnosis, 80
  for alcoholism diagnosis, 114
  for anxiety diagnosis, 52
  for conduct disorders, 164–165
  for depression diagnosis, 42–43
  for grand mal epilepsy diagnosis, 74
  for hyperactivity, 146–147
  for mental retardation diagnosis, 196
  for organic brain syndrome diagnosis, 61–63
  for performance anxiety, 173
  for psychosis diagnosis, 97–99
  for separation anxiety, 177
  for suicide risk assessment, 88–89

Rapport, 8
Reading disorders, 156–158
Relaxation exercises, 54, 56–57
Religion
  communication affected by, 11, 13
  in mental status examination, 29
Religious delusions, 33
Repetitive movements of patients, 30

School phobia, 171, 176
Sedation, 93, 204
Seizures, 71–77, 81
Sensorium, 34–35
Separation anxiety
  clinical management of, 177–180
  clinical picture of, 171, 176
  diagnosis of, 176–177
Sexual behavior
  in adolescence, 26
  in adulthood, 26
  in childhood, history of, 25
  in depression diagnosis, 43
  in interview, 18–19
Silence in interview, 14, 15, 20
Sleeping patterns
  with anxiety, 52
  with depression, 41, 42
  history of, 25
  with performance anxiety, childhood, 172
Slow movements of patients, 30
Social anxiety, 172
Somatic delusions, 33

Stuttering
  clinical management of, 191
  clinical picture of, 189–191
  diagnosis of, 191
Suicidal tendencies
  age of onset of, possible, 126
  with alcoholism, 90, 111
  clinical picture of, 87
  depression and, 41, 43, 49
  diagnosis of, 87–90
  from drug intoxication, 90
  management of, 90–93
  mental status exam of thoughts of, 33
  from psychosis, 90
  sedation for, 93
  with tricyclic antidepressants, 204

Tardive dyskinesia, 205, 210
Temporal lobe epilepsy, 72
Thioridazine, 106, 212
Thought content
  in mental status examination, 32–33
  with psychosis, 96
Thought disorders, 95–106
Thought process
  in mental status examination, 30–32, 37
  with psychosis, 95
Tranquilizers, minor, 212–213
Transference, 8
Trazodone, 203
Tremors, 111, 115
Tricyclic antidepressants
  amitriptyline, 47–48, 203, 211
  change of, 204
  for depression, 47
  desipramine, 48, 203, 204, 208
  imipramine, 48–49, 184, 203, 204
  overdosage of, 205
  secondary and toxic effects of, 204–205
  trial period and follow-up with, 203
Trifluoperazine, 205, 206, 207, 209
Trihexylphenidyl, 106, 213
Trust, 8

Visual hallucinations, 34, 67, 111
Vitamin deficiencies
  with alcoholism, 117
  in organic brain syndrome, 66, 67

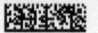